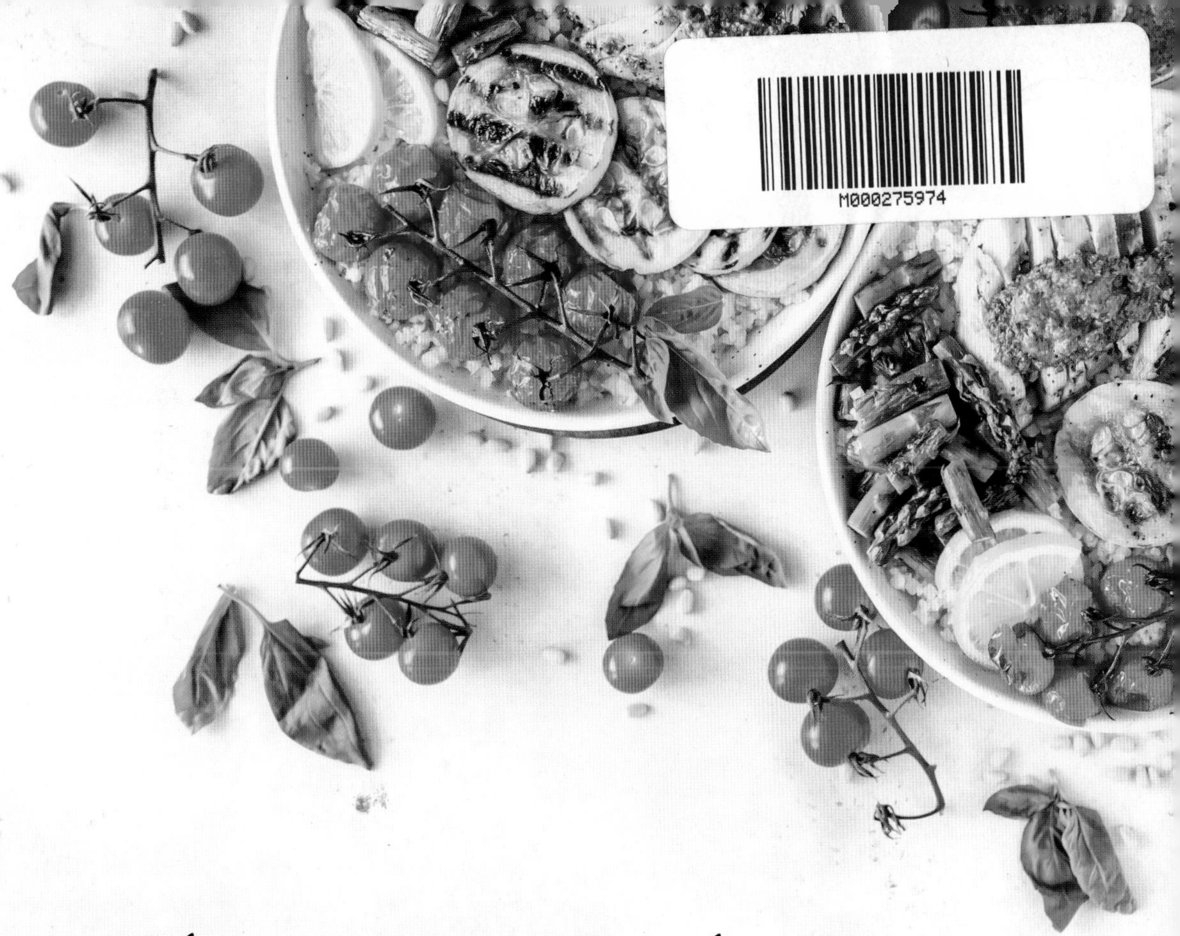

Clean Paleo
FAMILY COOKBOOK

100 DELICIOUS SQUEAKY CLEAN PALEO AND KETO RECIPES
TO PLEASE EVERYONE AT THE TABLE

Ashley McCrary
Creator of *Healthy Little Peach*

FAIR WINDS

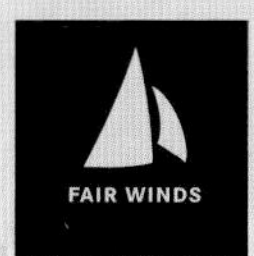

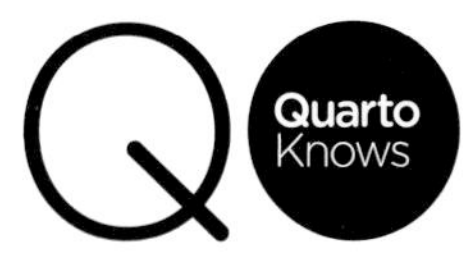

First Published in 2020 by Fair Winds Press, an imprint of The Quarto Group, 100 Cummings Center, Suite 265-D, Beverly, MA 01915, USA. T (978) 282-9590 F (978) 283-2742 QuartoKnows.com

Fair Winds Press titles are also available at discount for retail, wholesale, promotional, and bulk purchase. For details, contact the Special Sales Manager by email at specialsales@quarto.com or by mail at The Quarto Group, Attn: Special Sales Manager, 100 Cummings Center, Suite 265-D, Beverly, MA 01915, USA.

23 22 21 4 5

ISBN: 978-1-59233-910-5

Digital edition published in 2020
eISBN: 978-1-63159-787-9

Library of Congress Cataloging-in-Publication Data

Names: McCrary, Ashley, author.
Title: Clean paleo family cookbook : 100 delicious squeaky clean paleo and keto recipes to please everyone at the table / Ashley McCrary, creator of Healthy Little Peach.
Description: Beverly : Fair Winds Press, 2020. | Includes index.
Identifiers: LCCN 2019050194 (print) | LCCN 2019050195 (ebook) | ISBN 9781592339105 (trade paperback) | ISBN 9781631597879 (ebook)
Subjects: LCSH: High-protein diet--Recipes. | Prehistoric peoples--Nutrition. | Gluten-free diet--Recipes. | Ketogenic diet. | Pressure cooking. | Electric cooking, Slow. | LCGFT: Cookbooks.
Classification: LCC RM237.55 .M33 2020 (print) | LCC RM237.55 (ebook) | DDC 641.5/638–dc23
LC record available at https://lccn.loc.gov/2019050194
LC ebook record available at https://lccn.loc.gov/2019050195

Design and page layout: Laura Shaw Design, Inc.
Food photography: Ashley McCrary
Lifestyle photography: Beth Solano

Printed in China

The information in this book is for educational purposes only. It is not intended to replace the advice of a physician or medical practitioner. Please see your health-care provider before beginning any new health program.

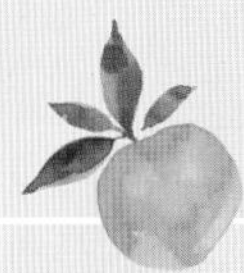

This book is dedicated to one of the loves of my life, Grandmother Sue Sue, who taught me to love my kitchen and to make a mess creating delicious meals for my family. It is also dedicated to the other loves of my life, my husband, Joel, and my two girls, Eloise and Eleanor. You guys make life easy, and I am so lucky that you are all mine.

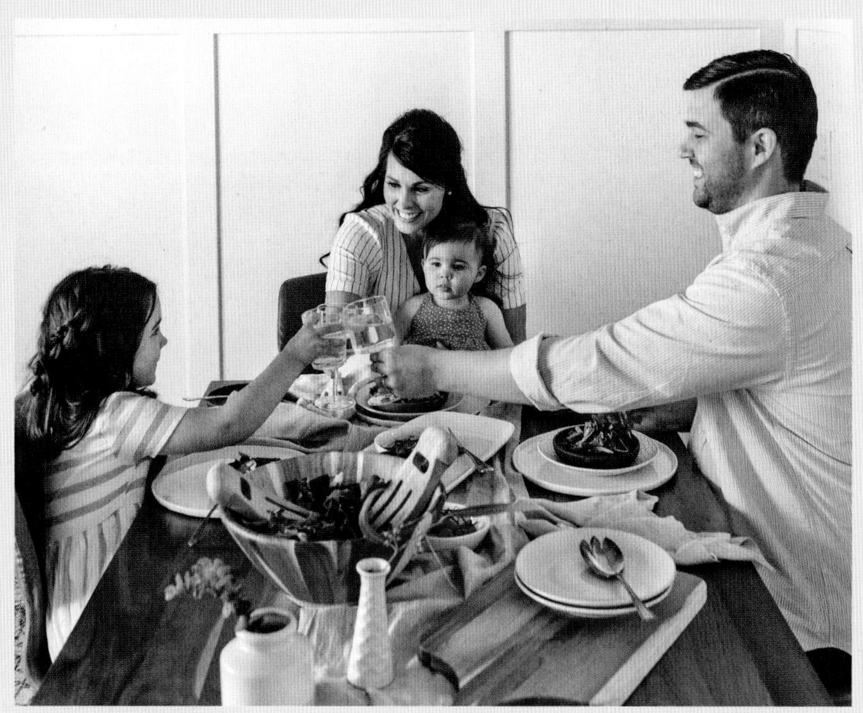

Foreword

As a lifelong foodie, I was delighted when Ashley asked me write the foreword for her cookbook, *Clean Paleo Family Cookbook*. Even though I have written a cookbook, I don't consider myself a writer–but I sure do love to cook and eat! I am excited when I discover a user-friendly cookbook filled with the kinds of recipes I enjoy the most–food that brings family and friends to the table. Ashley and I have known each other since she asked me for a bit of Instagram mentoring a couple years ago, and I quickly fell in love with her no-nonsense, generous heart and her engaging Southern drawl. Her Instagram Stories are approachable, and she shares her life from such a soulful place that you just can't help but watch. I love how she is always getting her family involved.

My level of enthusiasm for her winning combination of adult- *and* kid-friendly dishes could not be higher. As a mother, I know how tempting it is to want to make a separate meal for the kids. Ashley has made this extra effort unnecessary by creating dishes that are both nutritious and delicious–no one will even notice that they are squeaky clean! That is part of the beauty of this collection of recipes. Healthy family food that is delicious!

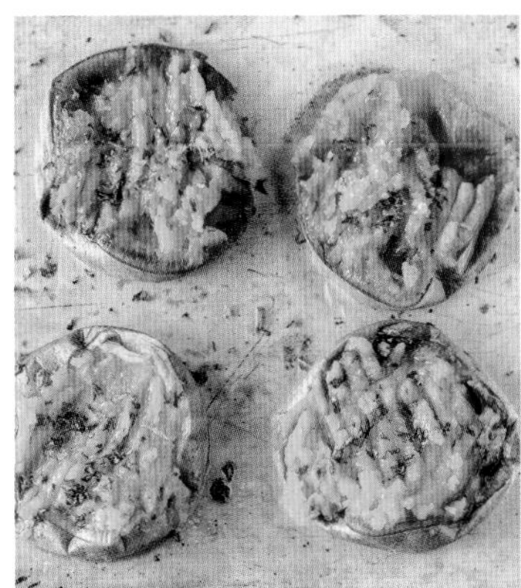

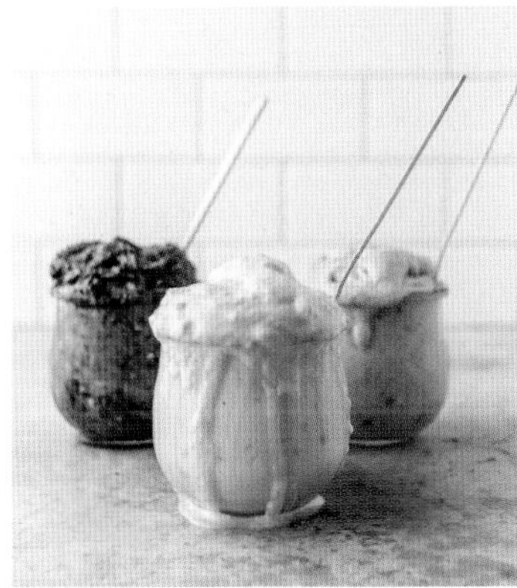

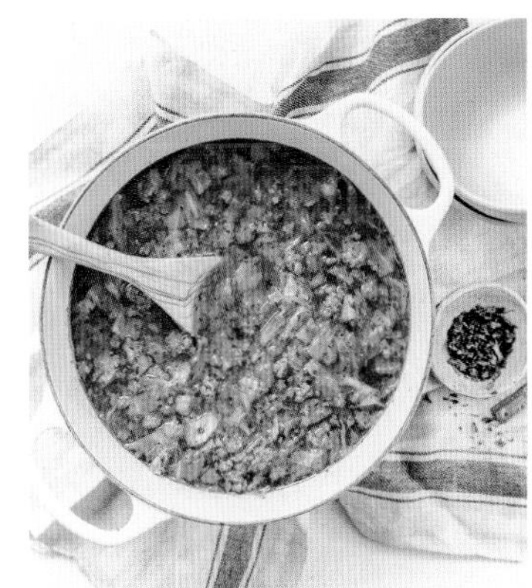

This cookbook makes cooking fun, sustainable, and enjoyable. My favorite cookbooks have comments and fingerprints and spills on the pages. They are used and loved. I suspect this cookbook will be one of those, especially when it comes to the Grilled Pork Chops with Peach Vinaigrette and the Philly Not So Cheesesteak Stuffed Peppers. I think of Ashley's dishes as comfort food made healthful. Her recipes will leave you feeling satisfied and content–and isn't that what we all want from a meal?

Teri Turner,

best-selling author of
No Crumbs Left

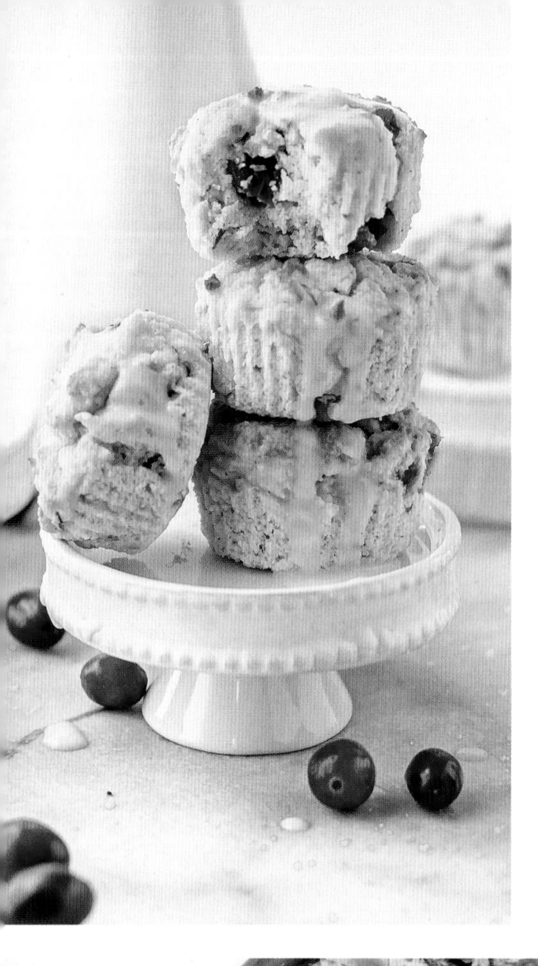
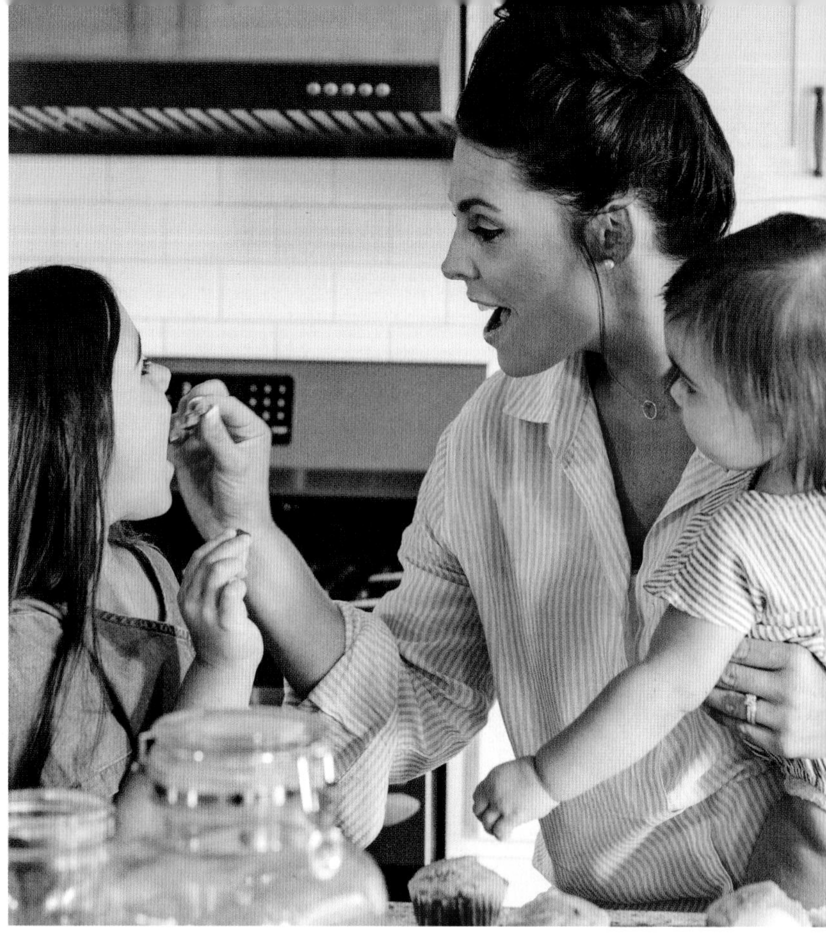
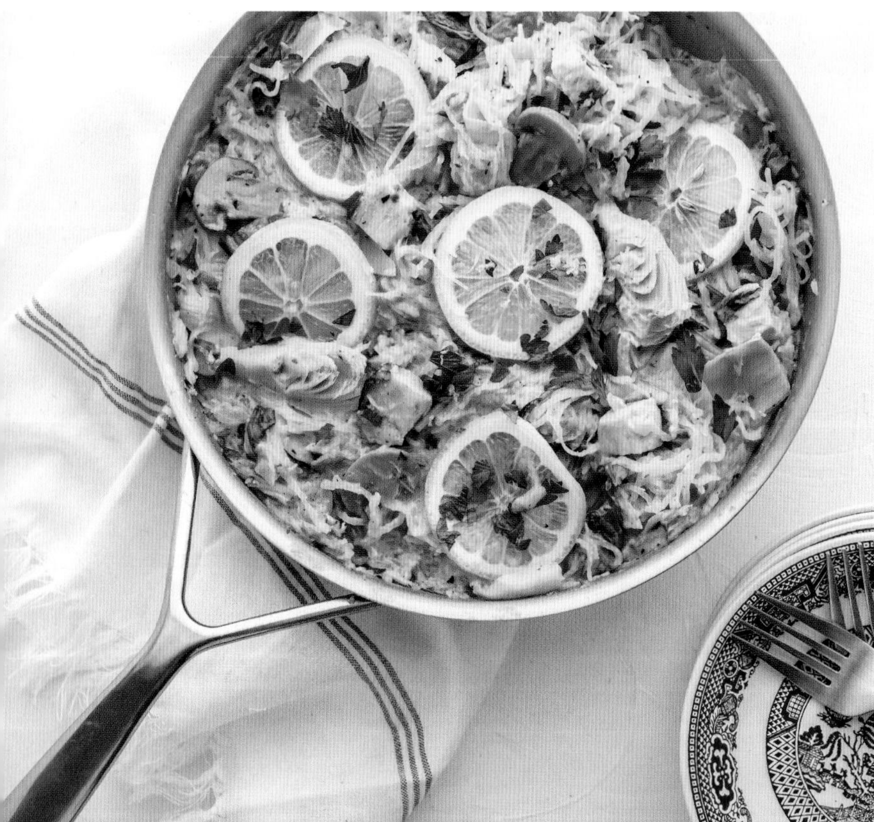
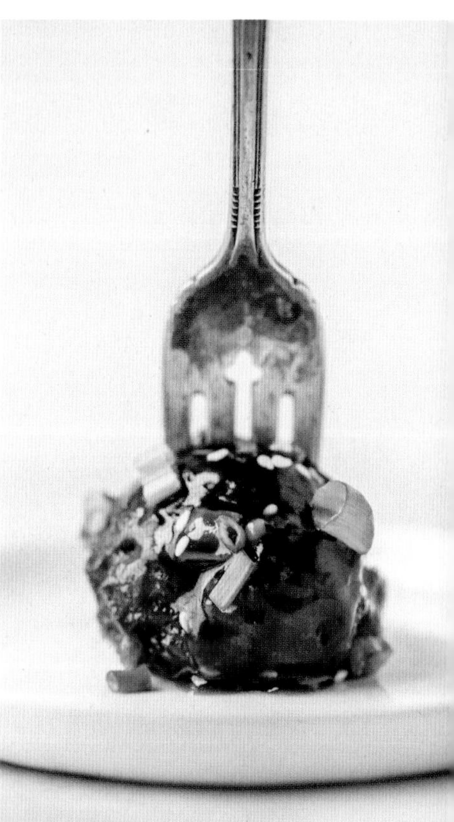

Contents

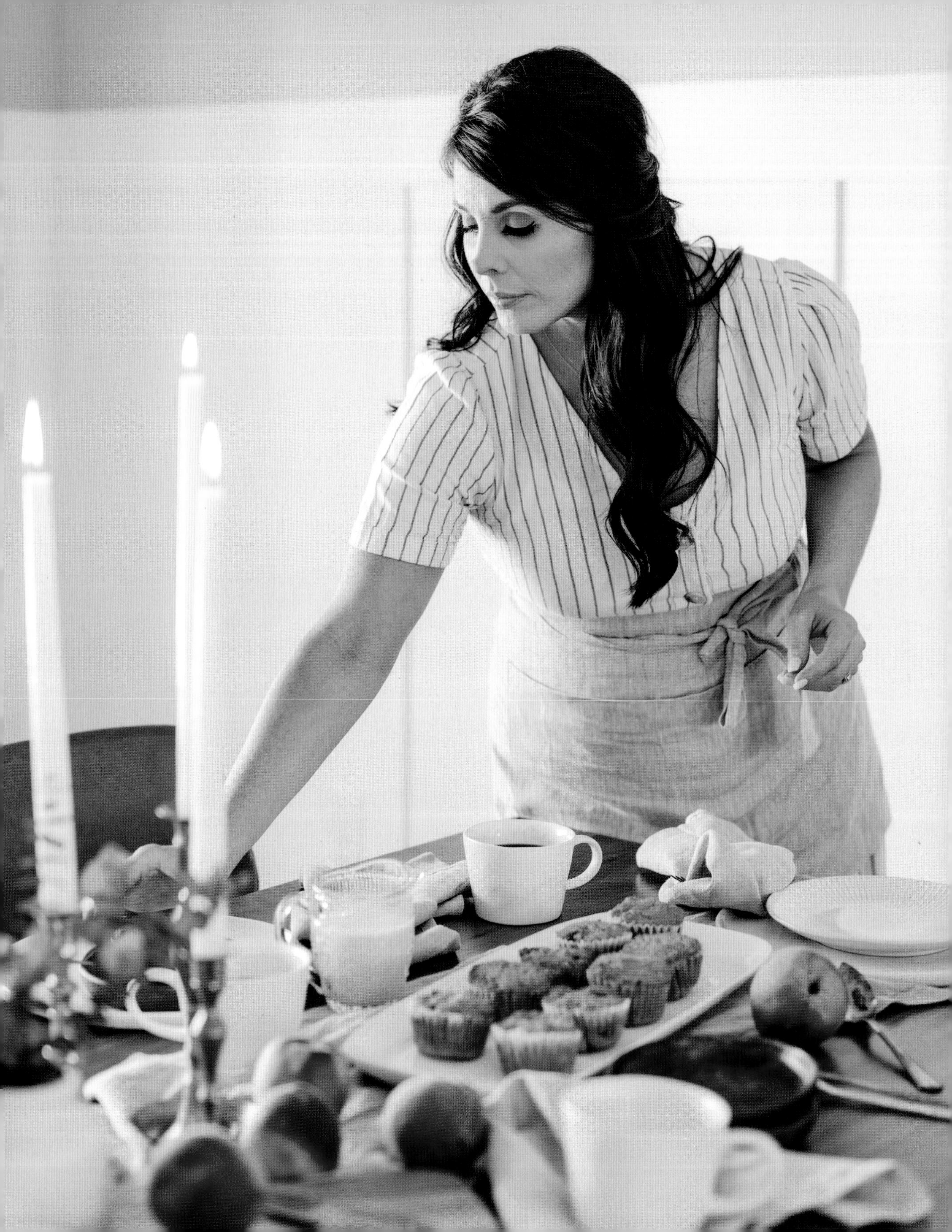

Introduction

Welcome to *The Clean Paleo Family Cookbook*! My name is Ashley McCrary, creator and recipe developer at Healthy Little Peach, a health and lifestyle blog. In addition, I am a wife to an amazing man, Joel, and mother to two beautiful girls, Eloise and Eleanor. In our cozy home, we create the best memories around the kitchen table. Our family strives to live the Paleo lifestyle, balanced with the occasional indulgent treat. I'm so passionate about sharing how the whole family can live a healthy life in a delicious and satisfying way. I have experienced firsthand how eating high-quality food can change your life and habits in a positive way.

My Story

Before switching to this lifestyle, I had battled eating disorders, body dysmorphia, depression, yo-yo dieting, and self-hate throughout most of my life. Additionally, I have been a polycystic ovarian syndrome (PCOS) fighter for years and struggled to get pregnant. My health was deteriorating by the day, and food was the only comfort I found. I began to lose myself and slip into a dark and unkind place.

I was extremely overweight and felt worthless as a woman. Finally, on a sunny December day in 2013, my tears turned to joy and we found out we were expecting our first baby girl, sweet Eloise. I was determined to make a life change not only for myself but also for my family. I remember at one point, as I caught a glimpse of my imperfect body in the mirror, I tore myself apart with the most hateful words as tears poured. As I stood there destroying myself, it came to me that if I couldn't love myself, then there was no way I could love my daughter and husband the way God intended. They needed a whole momma and wife, not a broken one.

A couple of days later, I found the Whole30 program, a 30-day reset challenge created by Melissa Hartwig Urban, and it completely changed my life. I dropped 80 pounds through sixteen rounds and found a new love and relationship with food. Today, I am no longer struggling with my PCOS symptoms and we were able to conceive a second child with no problems at all.

A New Life

Living Paleo cured what medication couldn't and healed and transformed my body and mind. It has taught me how to not only love food, but also most importantly, to love myself and my life. Before finding this lifestyle, I had been completely broken for years, and I truly believe it saved me.

Living this lifestyle has allowed me to find mental peace and clarity surrounding food. For years I lived with "food bondage" and extreme guilt surrounding all things food related. Switching to Paleo has allowed me to grow in my relationship with food and given me the confidence to raise my girls to value the importance of living a healthy lifestyle. I want them to truly enjoy the foods they choose to eat. My goal as their mother is to set the foundation and to supply them with the knowledge necessary to make their own healthy choices in the future.

I am passionate about sharing my journey and showing that the food we eat has a direct effect on our physical and mental well-being. Through my hardships, I have learned so much about who I truly am and what I am capable of. And if I can change, so can you. Be positive through your journey and have a purpose behind your change. Without purpose, it becomes just another diet that will more than likely fail. Stay consistent and give yourself and your family grace. In life, the more consistent we are with something, the more it becomes a routine. It is all a process and learning experience that takes time.

Through grace, time, and experience, it is my hope that healthy living will lead you not only to better physical health, but also to better mental health. For me, once I got the hang of living this way, my marriage grew, my friendships improved, and my soul felt more at peace. Through change, I became a whole person instead of living in a shell of sadness. Change can be hard, and it can take many days of starting over and making mistakes before you get it right. Hey, that's okay. It's worth it to start over and you are worth fighting for. Do it for your family, but better yet, do it for you.

Change Starts in the Kitchen

There is something extremely magical and heartwarming about sitting around the dining room table and eating a meal together as a family. Some of my best memories from childhood have a direct correlation with food and family. I remember the way my mother's and grandmother's meals would make me feel. If I was sad, my mom would whip up her famous beef stroganoff and veggies to warm my heart. If I was sick, her potato soup would soothe my tummy. And anytime I walked into Grandmother Sue Sue's house, she would poke her head out from her kitchen and say, "What can I make you to eat, baby?" Her love language was food, and she held my hand, pulled up a stool next to her stove, and taught me how to cook. She cooked with so much love and passion that I knew from a young age that I wanted to be just like her when I grew up.

Even though I will never come close to being half the cook my Sue Sue was, I am still following her direction and cooking from the heart. I can still picture her standing in her worn and food-stained apron, preparing some of her memorable chicken salad and licking her fingers to make sure it tasted just right. Isn't it special how food can vividly take you back to a specific time and place in your life? Now that I am a mother and a wife, I keep those memories close to my heart and have the same goal to create meals that leave a lasting impression on my family's hearts and tummies. My hopes are that this cookbook will take your hand and guide you in creating precious memories and meals with your family in a healthy and meaningful way.

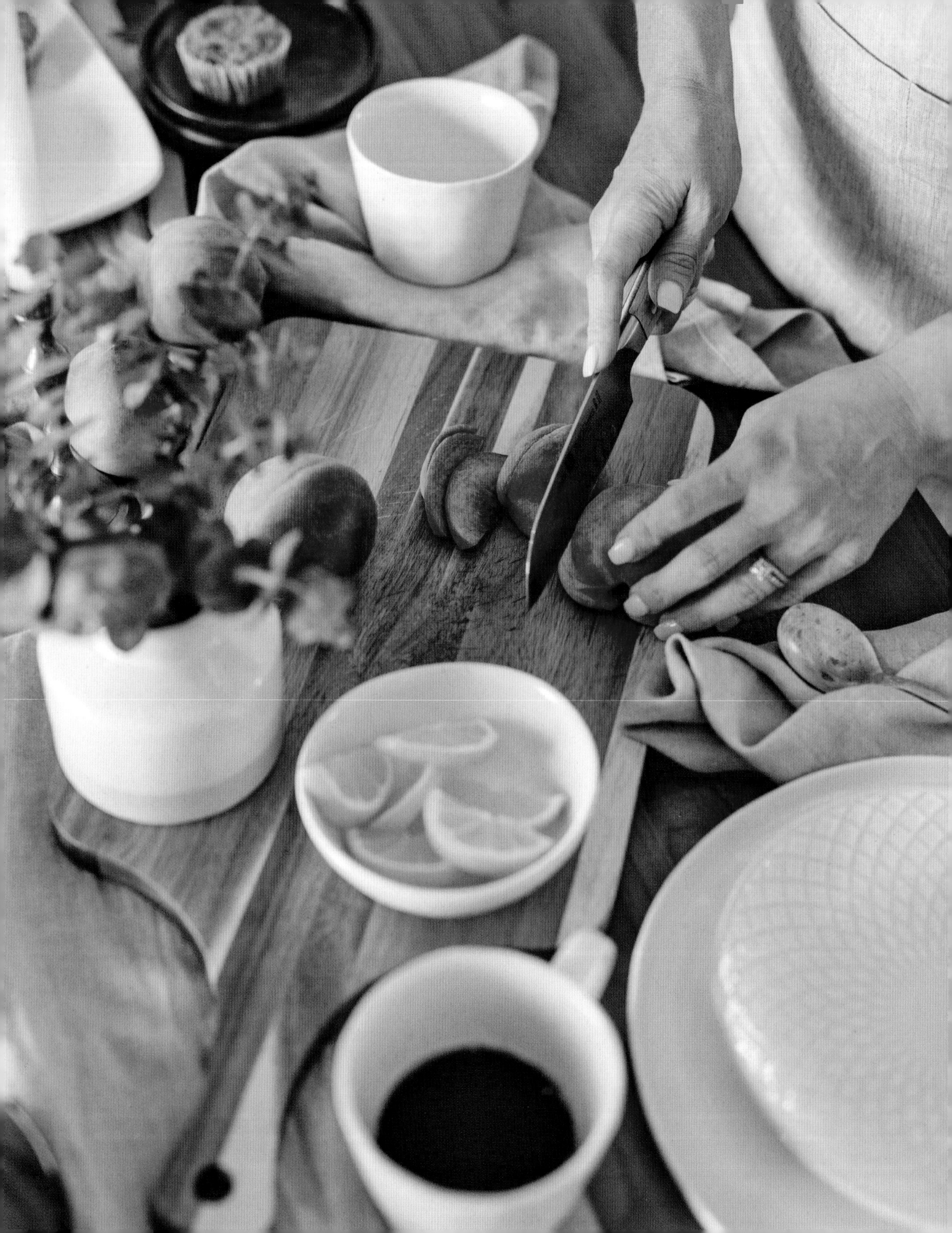

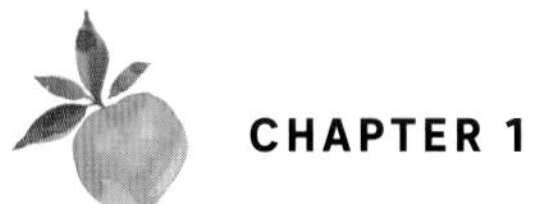

CHAPTER 1

What is Clean Paleo?

Since switching to the Paleo lifestyle, I have created many delicious recipes that make healthy living both easy and enjoyable. The purpose behind *The Clean Paleo Family Cookbook* is to support your journey in serving your whole family high-quality, healthy meals that will keep them satisfied–without breaking the bank. "Healthy" does not have to be boring, expensive, or tasteless!

Recipes Guidelines

Each of the recipes in this cookbook was designed around the Paleo diet. The idea behind Paleo eating comes from our hunter-gatherer ancestors and what they ate thousands of years ago. It's based on eating whole, unrefined, and unprocessed foods.

To help you on your healthy-eating journey, I've labeled each recipe with the following:

TRADITIONAL PALEO Contains NO grains, legumes, dairy, wheat, soy, gluten, or artificial ingredients. Only all-natural sweeteners such as raw honey, coconut sugar, real maple syrup, monk fruit, stevia extract, and erythritol. This way of eating is ideal for everyday life. Feel free to incorporate baked goods and treats on occasion.

SQUEAKY CLEAN PALEO Same as Traditional Paleo but without sweeteners, artificial or natural, apart from dates. Think of eating as cleanly as possible, excluding all desserts and treats. Use this as a guideline to establish better eating habits.

KETO PALEO Same as Traditional Paleo, except fewer carbs—there are no starchy veggies such as sweet potatoes. Compliant sweeteners include monk fruit, stevia extract, and erythritol.

FOODS TO EAT ON THE PALEO DIET

* **Meat:** Beef, lamb, chicken, turkey, pork, and game meats.
* **Seafood:** Salmon, trout, haddock, scallops, shrimp, shellfish, sardines, anchovies, and tuna.
* **Eggs:** Free-range, pastured, or omega-3-enriched eggs.
* **Vegetables:** Broccoli, cauliflower, kale, peppers, onions, carrots, radishes, tomatoes, zucchini, squash, salad greens, cucumbers, green beans, snow peas, snap peas, etc.
* **Fruits:** Apples, bananas, oranges, pears, avocados, berries, melons, and pineapple, etc.
* **Tubers:** Sweet potatoes, yams, turnips, and beets (but stay away from white potatoes).
* **Nuts and seeds:** Almonds, macadamia nuts, walnuts, hazelnuts, sunflower seeds, pumpkin seeds, pecans, cashews, and flax seeds.
* **Healthy fats and oils:** Extra virgin olive oil, light olive oil, coconut oil, avocado oil, sesame oil, and ghee.
* **Spices:** Sea salt, fresh and dried herbs and spices such as garlic, turmeric, rosemary, basil, oregano, dill, ground mustard seed, paprika, chili powder, and more.
* **Flours:** Almond, coconut, cassava, hazelnut, and plantain flours along with arrowroot starch/flour and tapioca starch/flour.

FOODS TO AVOID ON THE PALEO DIET

* **Sugar and high-fructose corn syrup:** Soft drinks, fruit juices, table sugar, candy, pastries, ice cream, and any other form of highly processed and sugary treat.
* **Grains:** Breads, pastas, and cereals made with wheat, spelt, rye, barley, oat, rice, and corn.
* **Legumes:** Beans (except for green beans), soybeans, chickpeas, peas (except for snow

and snap peas), black-eyed peas, peanuts, and lentils.

* **Dairy:** Avoid dairy, especially low fat (though some versions of Paleo do include full-fat dairy like grass-fed ghee).

* **Some oils:** Soybean oil, sunflower oil, cottonseed oil, corn oil, grapeseed oil, and safflower oil.

* **Trans fats:** Found in margarine and various processed foods. Usually referred to as "hydrogenated" or "partially hydrogenated" oils.

* **Artificial sweeteners:** Aspartame, sucralose, cyclamates, saccharin, and acesulfame potassium. Use natural sweeteners instead.

* **Highly processed foods:** Anything labeled "diet" or "low fat" or that has many additives.

Paleo Pantry and Kitchen Essentials

My promise with this cookbook is that switching your family to the Paleo lifestyle won't break your budget. It *is* going to cost a little bit up front, though, as you acquire all the healthy staple ingredients you're going to need to cook amazing dishes at the drop of a hat. And once you've mastered meal planning and prepping (see page 18), you won't go over budget.

PALEO PANTRY ESSENTIALS

Below are my favorite Paleo pantry items. Remember to read labels before purchasing to make sure the products comply with the guidelines of the diet you are following. (This goes for all products, not just those listed here.) Avoid any and all kinds of chemicals and added sugars.

Coconut aminos: Great to use as a soy sauce alternative. Perfect for stir-fry dishes, marinades, and sauces.

Paleo-compliant sweeteners:

* Honey (Traditional Paleo)

* Maple syrup (Traditional Paleo)

* Monk fruit (Keto and Traditional Paleo)

* Stevia (Keto and Traditional Paleo)

* Erythritol (Keto and Traditional Paleo)

* Dates (Squeaky Clean and Traditional Paleo)

Tapioca flour and arrowroot powder: Use these two starches to thicken glazes, sauces, gravies, and baked goods. Both have very little taste and won't affect the flavors in a recipe.

Ghee: Ghee is clarified butter that can be used just like regular butter. Use grass-fed ghee as your main cooking fat. While ghee is dairy, it's okay for paleo because it has been clarified.

Olive oils (extra virgin and extra light): Extra virgin olive oil is great to use for sautéing, and the extra light or light olive oil is a must-have when making sauces and dressings. It's the main ingredient in most of the sauce recipes in this cookbook. Never use regular olive oil when making sauces, as they will come out thin and bitter.

Coconut oil: Used as a cooking fat and in many Paleo baked goods. Unrefined coconut oil smells like coconuts but doesn't taste like them.

Compliant cooking spray: Cooking spray is a must for coating skillets, pans, and baking sheets to prevent sticking. Avocado and olive oil cooking sprays are my favorites. Be sure to select pump sprays and not aerosol, which can contain noncompliant ingredients.

Nutritional yeast: Nutritional yeast has a nutty, almost cheesy texture and taste, making it ideal to use as a cheese substitute on eggs and roasted veggies. Look for nutritional yeast flakes, not brewer's yeast.

Coconut and almond flours: Both are a great substitute for regular wheat flour and can be used in savory dishes and baked goods. These flours can also be used as a thickening agent.

Vinegars: In many Paleo recipes, you'll find apple cider vinegar, rice vinegar, balsamic vinegar, and red wine vinegar, which add great flavors. All these vinegars are Paleo friendly. Just avoid malt vinegar, which may contain gluten.

Hot sauce: Find your compliant favorite, as it's a great way to add flavor to any dish. I love incorporating it into soups and casseroles and using it on top of eggs.

Nut butters: Almond, cashew, and pecan butters are great for snacks and can also add flavor to Paleo Asian-inspired dishes.

85% (or darker) chocolate and unsweetened cocoa powder: Great for baking! The darker, the better.

Canned goods:

* Diced, crushed, and whole tomatoes
* Tomato paste
* Tomato sauce (no sugar added)
* Tuna fish
* Salmon
* Coconut milk (unsweetened, full fat)
* Black olives

Seasoning: Seasonings add a ton of flavor to recipes. Again, be sure to read the labels for sneaky ingredients such as added sugar and chemicals.

Ground mustard: This is an ingredient used as an acidic component in a lot of Paleo recipes. Most commonly used in things such as spice rubs, salad dressings, and soups.

Xanthan gum: Can be used as a thickening agent for Keto Paleo recipes as it has fewer carbs.

Gelatin: Can be used as a thickening agent in Keto Paleo sauces and soups and is even found in some Paleo baking recipes.

KITCHEN ESSENTIALS

Below are my recommendations for kitchen tools and essentials that will make Paleo cooking a breeze. These are just recommended and not required to live a Paleo lifestyle.

Electric pressure cooker: This little magical gadget makes life so much easier after a busy day. It will cook just about anything in warp speed. It makes a busy life and healthy living much more manageable. It's also useful for the recipes in chapter 7.

Slow cooker: Great for throwing in a roast, a whole chicken, soup, or stew on a lazy Sunday or before work in the morning. Also useful for recipes in chapter 7.

Air fryer: This may be my all-time favorite kitchen gadget. Just like the electric pressure cooker, it cooks things extremely quickly using hot air and no added fat. We love using it for chicken breast tossed with almond flour–it makes the perfect healthy crispy tenders, like those on page 154.

Immersion blender: A must-have for making mayonnaise, sauces, and creamy soups.

Wide-mouth mason jars: These are amazing to make your sauces in and store for the week. I also love using them to store soups and leftovers.

Glass meal-prep containers: Great for meal prep and storing leftovers.

Instant-read thermometer: Buying one of these is one of the best investments you can make. It will help make sure that your meats are cooked to the proper temperature.

Milk frother: A frother adds a coffee shop feel to your morning coffee. Use your favorite nut milk, and it will give your regular cup of joe a frothy, latte-style feel.

Food processor: You can shred or chop large amounts of veggies and protein in a food processor. Also great for making homemade sauces and nut butters.

Dutch oven: Dutch ovens are perfect for making soups, stews, and even whole chickens and roasts. They can go from the stove top, to the oven, to the table, making them a good option if you don't own a slow cooker.

Regular or high-speed blender: Great for making soups, smoothies, and cauliflower mash.

Menu Planning and Meal Prepping

Menu planning and meal prepping is key when living a healthy lifestyle. Being organized and prepared are extremely important. Just think how easy it is to order takeout or boil up a pound of pasta when you walk into your kitchen at 6:00 p.m. and have no idea what you want to make for dinner. Well, healthy living *can* be just as easy—if you are prepared and ready.

Plan one day a week where you can get in the kitchen and prep a few different meal options, which will reduce stress during the rest of the week. Don't overcomplicate the process. I like to prep a few different lunch and breakfast options, but not go overboard. In addition, I like to cook a few proteins and roast up a few veggie options. That way, I can build different meals with what I already have cooked in the fridge.

In addition, have a menu on your refrigerator that you build weekly. Once you have it written out, check your freezer and fridge and make sure you have all the ingredients necessary to execute your meals during the week. If not, make a list and hit the grocery store and get prepared. Here are some other ideas to get you started.

KEEP IT SIMPLE

If you're already living a busy life, overcomplicating the process of *healthy* living can really sabotage your chances of success. Make sure you are building your meals in a simple way. Build your plate with mostly veggies, a serving of protein and fat, and add in the occasional fruit serving. I often add my sauces (found in chapter 1) to help liven up plain veggies or protein. For example, I'll prepare Mac's Awesome Sauce (page 31) or Chili Lime Sauce (page 32) to add flavor to chicken breasts or Brussels sprouts. The sauces totally transform the flavors in a healthy way, and I allow them to count as a fat serving.

DON'T OVERPREP

I have found that overprepping meals will actually cost more money. I'm the type of person who will get sick of eating the same thing over and over, so I refuse to make a giant batch of one or two things and expect to eat that in four or five different meals. I'll end up throwing them away by week's end because I get burned out so quickly. The only time I will cook a full dish is for breakfasts. I tend to make a frittata on Sunday that will serve for a few breakfast or lunch meals during the week.

TRY "BUFFET-STYLE" MEAL PREP

My prep looks a little different than the traditional meal prep. I use the "buffet-style" prep where I cook a variety of proteins, veggies, and even some carbohydrates. I store them all in different glass containers and pull them when I need to build a meal. Using this method gives me more freedom in the meals I create and allows me to change things up in an easy and convenient way without getting bored.

For example, I usually cook two or three different proteins (say, chicken, ground beef, and steak) and roast a few different veggies (Brussels sprouts, butternut squash, zucchini). I can use chicken breast in salads, protein bowls, and even eggs, and I can alternate the veggies that I use for dinner. (I don't make any more beyond that or I'll get bored.) Additionally, my girls love eating sweet potatoes with their dinner throughout the week, so I will wrap four or five in aluminum foil and throw them in the slow cooker on Sunday afternoon, which will make weeknight dinners even easier.

LEFTOVERS SAVE LIVES

Another reason I don't make too many actual full dishes on Sundays is because I love making extra of whatever I'm cooking to use for the next day's leftovers. For example, if I make taco salad on Tuesday, I always make extra to take leftovers for lunch on Wednesday. By incorporating leftovers, it allows for less waste and easier options throughout the week.

Here are just a few examples of how you can transform prepared proteins and even full recipes into completely new dishes. You're only limited by your imagination.

Salsa Verde Chicken (page 143): Add on top of salads, stuff inside a lettuce wrap or avocado, or simply eat with a side of veggies.

Taco Meat (page 72) : Serve on top of cauliflower rice, on salads, or on top of plantain chips or tostones for quick nachos.

Chili (page 146) : Stuff in a sweet potato, top over clean hot dogs, or serve with plantain chips or tostones for nachos.

Shredded Pork (page 142) : Add on top of plantain chips or tostones for the perfect nacho option or turn into a power bowl using cauliflower rice and veggies as the base. Top with one of my yummy sauces, starting on page 27.

Sausage Skillet Stir-Fry (page 110): This dish serves as a great breakfast, lunch, or dinner. Top with Chili Lime Sauce (page 32) or Mac's Awesome Sauce (page 31), and this is a quick, complete meal.

Turkey Meatloaf Muffins (page 152): Though this recipe is included in the kid chapter, it's awesome for everyone in the family. These muffins work for any meal and can be served with a steamed veggie, sweet potato, or side salad to make a complete meal. They even make a perfect snack option.

Living Paleo on a Family Budget

People assume that eating Paleo is expensive. All that meat. None of the cheap "convenience" items. Over the years, I've worked hard to figure out how to get the most bang for the buck, especially when feeding a family. Here are some tips to help you on your Paleo journey.

1. MAKE A PLAN AND MENU AND STICK TO IT.

Planning takes time, but consistency is key. Planning out a menu not only allows you to stay on track, but it also helps save money because you're creating your grocery list in a more meaningful way.

First, build your meals around the budget you have set. I use Dave Ramsey's Envelope System (www.daveramsey.com), because it allows me to physically see how much money I have to spend on groceries. Plan your grocery trips every two weeks and make a detailed list that fits your menu. When shopping, buy exactly what's on your list and don't get sidetracked.

2. ASSESS WHAT YOU HAVE.

Keep an inventory of what is in your fridge and pantry. Before going to the grocery store, make sure to check your shopping list against your inventory. This will allow you to save some cash by not buying unneeded items.

This one tip has saved my budget more than any of the other tips. Before building my meal menus, I check my freezer, fridge, and pantry and build meals with what I have first. Then when I run out of things to make, I start building new meal ideas with things I need from the grocery store.

3. EAT MORE EGGS.

Allow eggs to be your main protein source a few times a week. Build casseroles, frittatas, or just make a big delicious breakfast for dinner. This tip will honestly save you so much money! To support you in this area, I have added a ton of egg recipes in the breakfast chapter that can be used for any meal.

4. SIMPLIFY AND REPEAT.

Repeating and using leftover meals will help you in your journey to healthy living. It's important to get into a routine by finding meals that you wouldn't mind repeating once a week. For example, I pick a day of the week—say, "Taco Salad Tuesdays"—and we'll do that every Tuesday for the month. To change things up, the next month we will pick another favorite cheap meal and repeat it every week for that month. My family looks forward to these days of the week because it becomes routine.

QUICK MEAL AND SNACK OPTIONS

Life can get extremely busy, and during those times, Unhealthy Eating Habits can rear its ugly head. Here are some at-a-glance ideas for what to make when you're short on time and need a quick and healthy meal or snack option.

BREAKFAST	LUNCH	DINNER	SNACKS
Frittata (page 60)	BLT lettuce wrap (butter lettuce wrap, bacon, tomato, and mayo)	Sausage Skillet Stir-Fry (page 110) over cauliflower rice	Apples with nut butter
Chicken Fajita Egg Cups (page 66)	Salsa Verde Chicken, Slow Cooker Version (page 143)	Pot Roast and Curry Coleslaw (page 144)	Veggies dipped in Ranch Dressing (page 30)
Scrambled eggs and bacon	Tuna Salad Stuffed Avocados	Steak and veggies (page 84)	Protein bars such as RBars, RXBARS, and Lärabars (read labels)
Breakfast salad of prosciutto, arugula, fried egg, olive oil	Protein with greens/ veggies	Sheet pan meals (such as on page 103)	Cashews, clean beef jerky
Chia seed pudding (page 68)	Taco salad (page 72)	Burger Bowls (page 136)	Chive and Onion Mixed Nuts (page 46)
2 boiled eggs and 1 cup (240 ml) bone broth	Chipotle chicken salad (page 77)	Soups (page 147 and 149)	Deviled eggs (page 51)
			Turkey Meatloaf Muffins (page 152)

Get Kids on Board for Healthy Living

Getting kids on a healthy eating path can be an extremely hard task. As parents, it is our job to do the work and set the foundation early; we need to be a positive role model and teacher. With health comes balance, and this must be the case with kids living a healthy lifestyle. Always offer your kids wholesome food choices and educate them on the importance of eating well. You should never feel like you have to make a separate meal every single night to please your kids. Simply re-create the meal you're already making in a more appealing and kid-friendly way (see page 151). Some nights are hard, and you'll want to give in and throw some frozen fish sticks and tater tots in the oven to satisfy them, but don't; stay consistent. Through consistency, my girls have come to embrace the Paleo lifestyle and truly love the food that I put on their plates.

Make sure you are still allowing your children the *occasional* treat. I have included some Paleo treat options in chapter 9 that serve as great desserts or occasional indulgences—not only for your kids, but for the whole family. Kids should never be deprived or made to feel guilty for craving treats. I always want my girls to enjoy mealtimes around the kitchen table and not dread coming together for a meal.

Remember, healthy kids grow up to be healthy adults.

TRANSFORM AN ADULT PLATE INTO A KID-FRIENDLY ONE

Dinnertime can become a real hassle when you have to make three different meals to please everyone at the table. In the past, my daughter Eloise would throw a fit for chicken nuggets and french fries. When I gave in, I ended up spending more time and money to make sure everyone had what they wanted.

When I came to the realization that I am not the mom who's going to spend hours in the kitchen and endless amounts of money at the grocery store, things changed for the better. I began making kid versions of the healthy meals I was already preparing. What does that mean? Ask yourself, "How can I present this plate so it's not overwhelming to a child?" Add a piece of fruit, put sauce on the side (or not at all), and even get your kids involved and allow them to pick out a veggie.

Slowly, Eloise began to love the idea of eating what her mommy and daddy were eating. I even let her get involved in the menu. I would give her choices as to what fruit she wanted, and she began to love the idea of helping build her plate.

ELOISE'S 5 TIPS FOR PALEO/HEALTHY EATING

Oh, the wisdom of children. At the tender age of five, sweet Eloise has her own ideas on how to eat so she can grow big and strong:

1. Eat a hard-boiled egg . . . or two.
2. Slap some fruit on it; add fruit as a dessert and make it fun.
3. Be sure to allow for treats every now and then. Pizza is tasty sometimes.
4. Kids should be able to help select and prepare meals.
5. Eat what your mommy and daddy put on your plate and smile about it.

EXAMPLES OF KID-FRIENDLY PLATED MEALS

Frittata with diced avocado, berries	Hamburger sliders with clean pickle slices and mustard, fruit, sliced avocado	Crispy chicken strips, carrots, and grapes
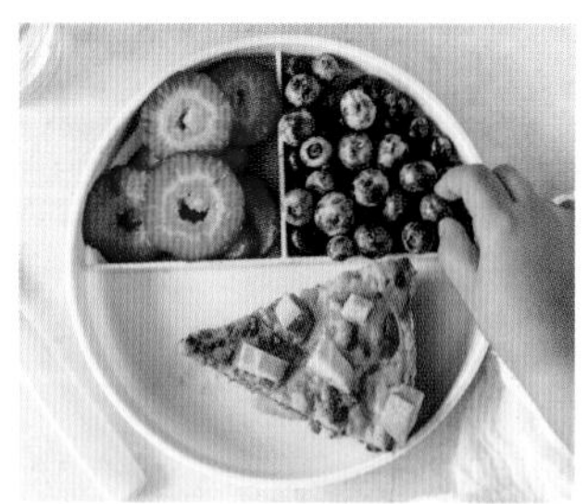	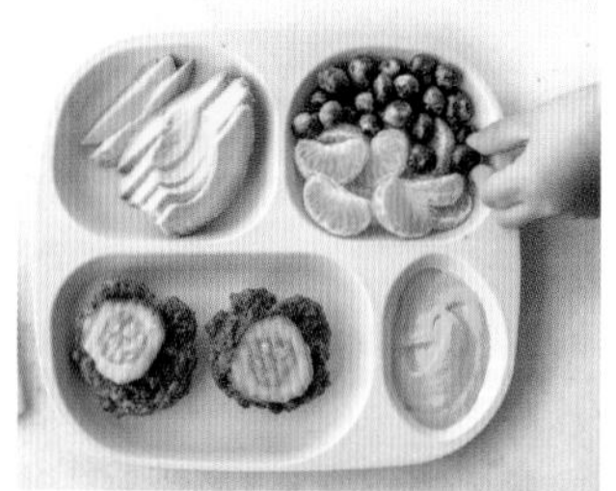	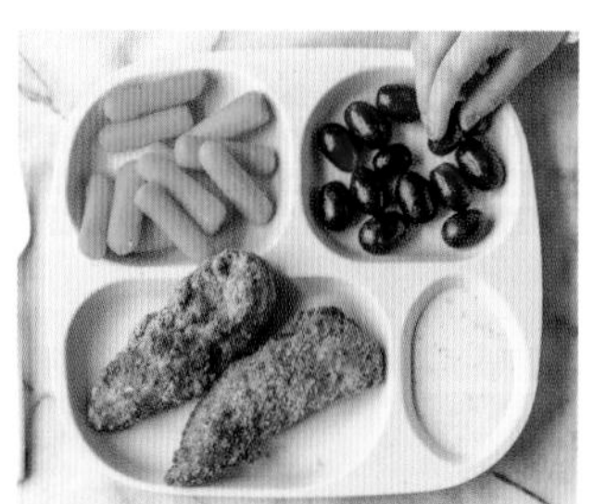
Scrambled eggs, a clean chopped hot dog, orange and apple slices	Turkey meatloaf muffins, diced sweet potatoes, grapes and strawberries	Sliced pork chop, sweet potato fries, cucumbers and ranch dressing, strawberries
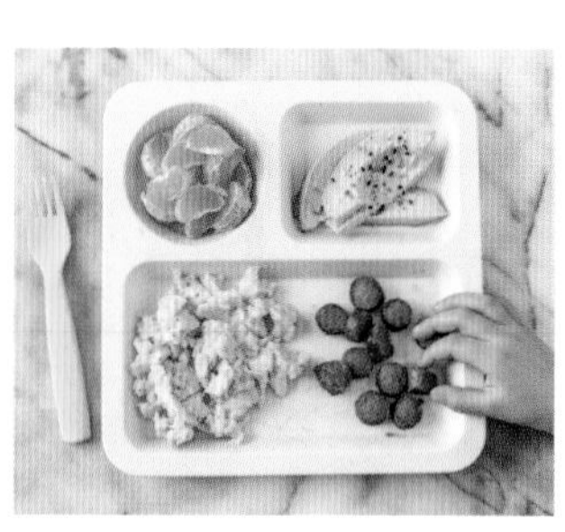	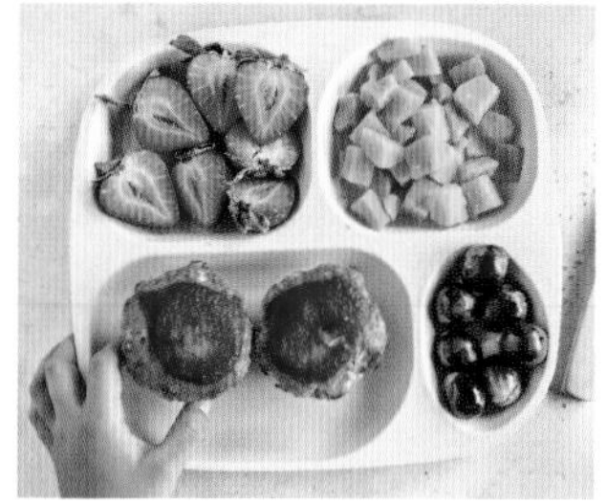	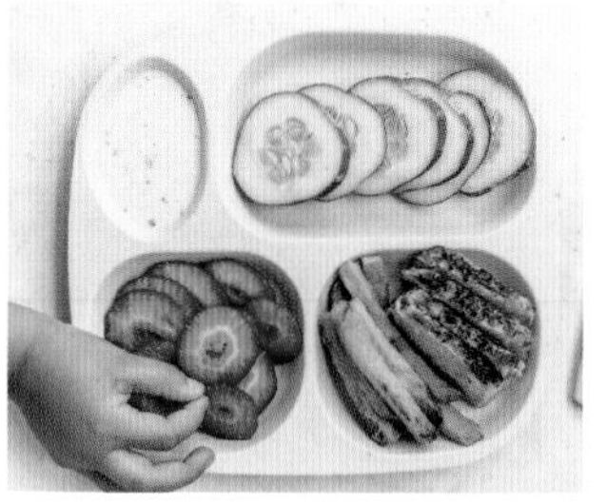

KID-FRIENDLY SNACK OPTIONS

- Chocolate-Covered Frozen Banana Bites (page 161)
- Mixed nuts with rolled-up clean lunch meat
- A hard-boiled egg with pineapple chunks or grapes
- Clean snack bars such as RBars, RXBARS, and Lärabars
- Apple “pizzas”: sliced apples topped with almond butter and fruit of choice

Mamma Bear Meal

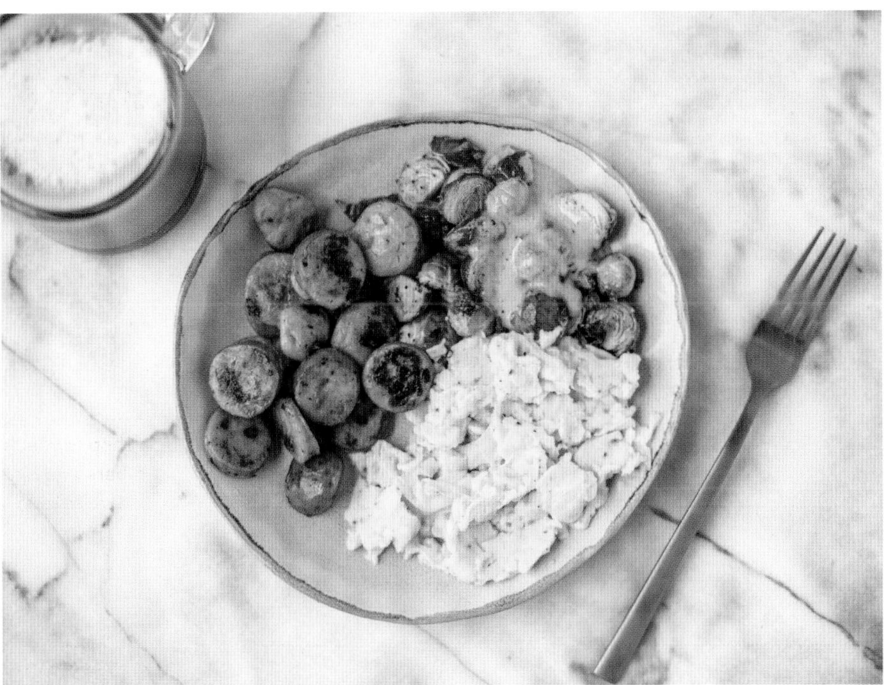

Baby Bear Meal

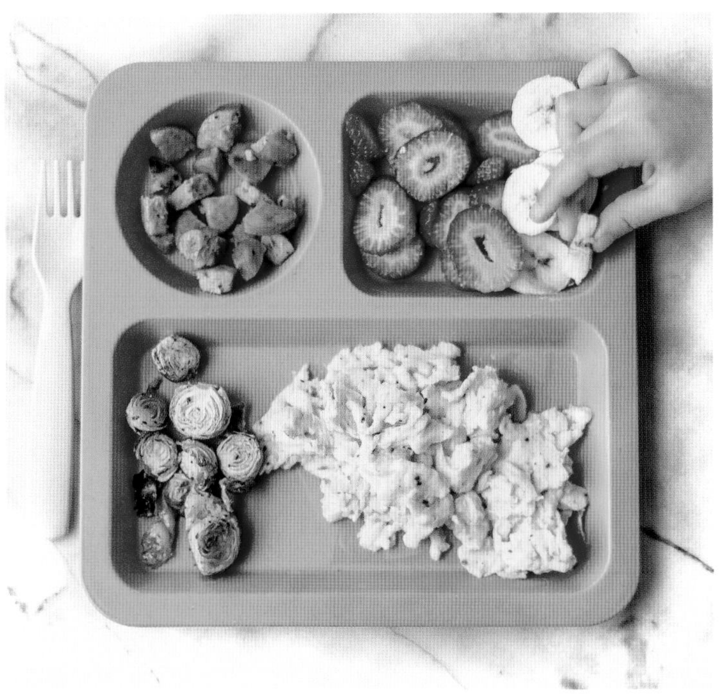

Healthy Family Living with a Busy Schedule

A lot of parents feel defeated by a busy schedule; I get it. But let's stop using this as the main excuse as to why we can't get healthy. Most families in the United States are in the same boat: There aren't enough hours in the day to get everything done, let alone find time to cook a healthy meal, right? But a busy life doesn't mean having to forego healthy eating habits. It simply requires some planning and setting boundaries for yourself and your family. Here are my four Big Tips to help you find balance and live a healthy and sustainable life.

BIG TIP #1: CLEAN YOUR HOUSE

A fresh mind equals a fresh life. Before starting a healthy lifestyle, fully commit and mentally prepare yourself for an overall lifestyle change, not only for yourself but for the whole family. The most important thing you can do at the beginning of every week is clean your house. Never start a week in chaos with a messy home, an unplanned menu, or unprepped food. Think *lifestyle* here; overall health has so many more components than the foods we consume. Clean your house, fridge, pantry, and, most of all, clean up that *attitude*!

BIG TIP #2: END KID DRAMA

"Too bad you want pizza instead of my beautiful cauliflower mash... You ain't getting it." (Drop the microphone.)

Boom. That's right: Kids don't make the rules. Your three-year-old child should not have power over what they are going to eat for dinner every single night. In the beginning of our journey of healthy living, my daughter Eloise would snarl at my Paleo creations, throw her body on the ground, and act like a total drama queen. She would insist on chocolate milk to wash down her chicken nuggets. She really lost her mind for about a week, but guess what happened after that? She realized that she didn't have the power over what she was going to eat. I refused to give in, and I won the battle. She ended up loving her carrot slices, chopped chicken with homemade ranch dressing, and of course her beloved blueberries. She got to the point where she'd ask for seconds.

Here's the problem: Parents get so busy in life, they look for shortcuts. Hey, I'm guilty of this too. But we're not doing our children a service by giving in to their demanding ways. Once you set boundaries and train your kids to choose healthy options, you are setting them up with the knowledge they need to make healthy choices of their own.

Offering children choices is a great way to make them think they are controlling the situation. I might say, "Hey, baby, do you want green beans or carrots with your chicken tonight?" She gets so excited that I am involving her in food choices that she'll sometimes ask if she can have both. Don't back down; involve your kids in their healthy food choices, and overall, *be the parent.* Don't use the phrase "my kid is a picky eater..." because they will start to catch on to the idea of what the expectations of healthy eating are—I promise.

BIG TIP #3:
SET A SCHEDULE AND STICK TO IT

It's so important to make a plan and write out a menu every week and stick to it. Sit down with your calendar and review what events you and your family have coming up and figure out how to incorporate healthy meal options during the busy times.

Map it out. Plan your shopping trips and meal preps around your schedule; in fact, pencil it into your calendar and make sure you are making it a priority. If you do this, come Monday when your kid has ballet or football practice, you won't be overwhelmed. You can designate that night for eating out at a healthy restaurant that offers Paleo dishes. Being prepared is going to make this process so much easier.

BIG TIP #4:
KEEP CALM AND MAKE A FRITTATA

This is the game changer, friends. You can't wake up on Monday morning and try to prep your family's breakfast, lunch, and dinner for the week. You will lose yo dang mind. So, always make a frittata on Sunday. Slice that beautiful pie into serving sizes and put them in a glass container. Pull it from the fridge in the mornings and quickly heat up. You not only have an easy meal, but it will fill you up, leaving you satisfied until lunch. Frittatas are so versatile and flavorful that they even serve as a great lunch or dinner. Check out my Red Pepper and Sausage Frittata on page 60 or toss in whatever cooked veggies you already have on hand.

Now let's see how easy—and delicious—it is to start eating healthy!

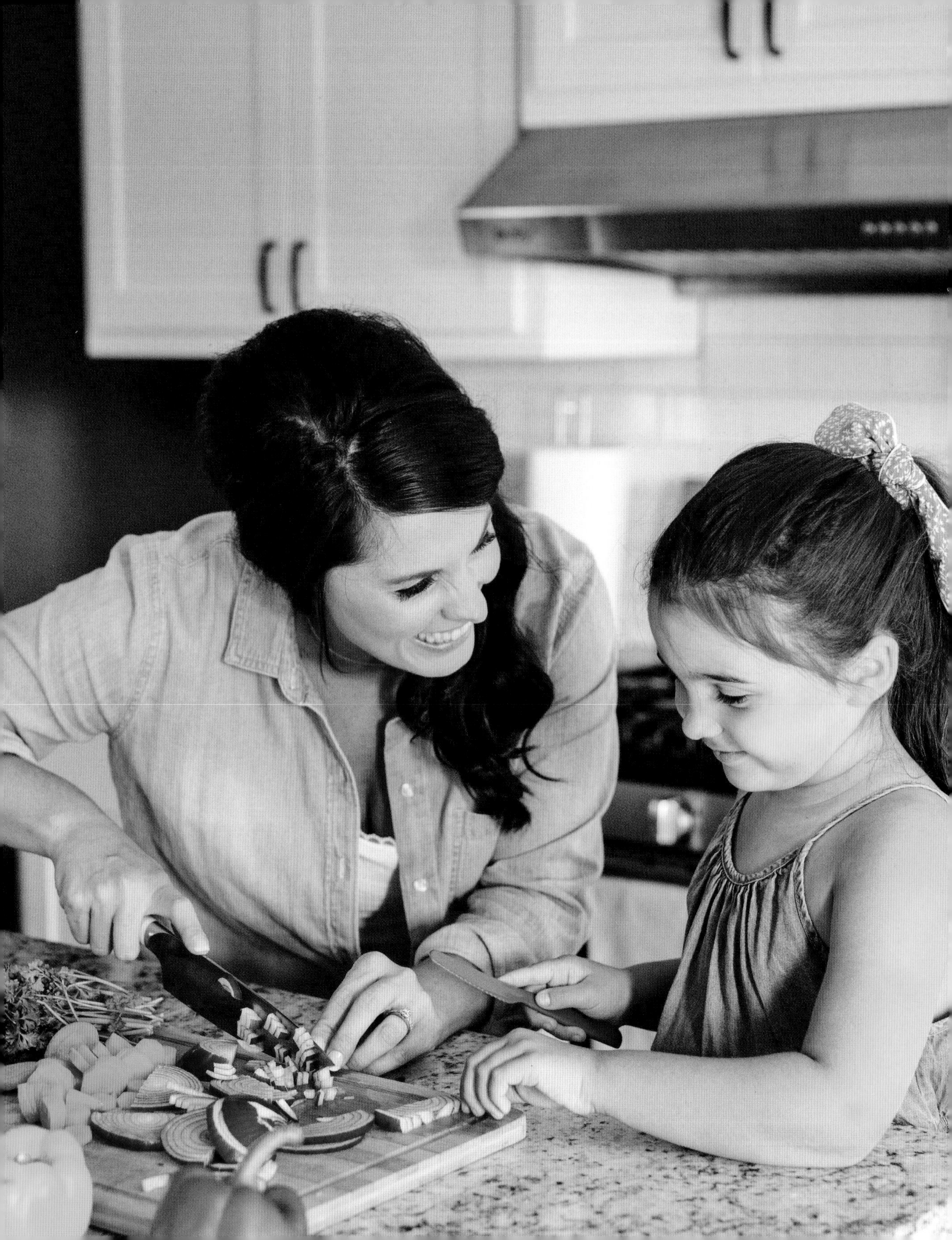

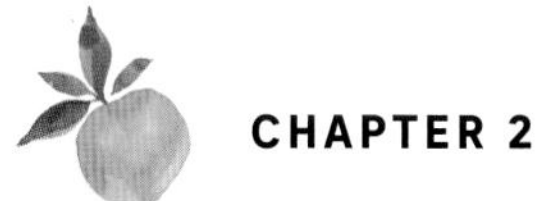

CHAPTER 2

Sauces and Appetizers

Sauces and dressings are by far some of my favorite recipes to create because they add amazing flavor and texture to any dish. In fact, I am known as the "Sauce Queen" because you can always find homemade sauces in my fridge and on my dinner plate. In this chapter, you'll find a few, like the Chili Lime Sauce (page 32) and Mac's Awesome Sauce (page 31), that are great with just about anything. I keep them on hand as part of my weekly meal prep. Others, like the Peach Vinaigrette (page 36) and the Basil Pesto (page 37), are good for building specific recipes, but they're so delicious you'll want to put them on everything.

Not only do sauces and dressings tickle my fancy, but appetizers just make me happy. They have so many uses, and they're just the cutest! I feel lavish when I line my kitchen counter with all sorts of fun finger foods. I've come up with some delicious recipes that will serve your next holiday party (Chili-Lime Deviled Eggs, page 51), tailgate (Buffalo, Dill, and Bacon Wings, page 44), or just a cozy family night (Asian Meatballs, page 42) in a yummy fashion. You can entertain the healthy, wholesome way, and your family and friends will never know.

Mayo

This classic condiment uses light olive oil blended with an egg to make a great base for a lot of dressings. It's so simple to prepare, you won't remember why you ever bought it in a jar. Note that this recipe uses a raw egg. If you have concerns about consuming raw eggs, use pasteurized eggs.

SQUEAKY CLEAN PALEO / KETO PALEO / TRADITIONAL PALEO

Makes: 1 cup (240 g) / **Prep Time:** 2 minutes / **Total Time:** 5 minutes

1 cup (240 ml) light olive oil
1 large egg
½ teaspoon ground mustard
½ teaspoon sea salt
½ teaspoon lemon juice

IMMERSION BLENDER VERSION

1. Add the olive oil, egg, mustard, salt, and lemon juice to a wide-mouth mason jar.
2. Place the immersion blender over the top of the egg and turn the blender to low speed. Leave the blender here and don't move it until the mixture begins to turn white.
3. Increase the speed and begin to slowly lift the blender stick up. Blend, taking the immersion blender up, down, and to the sides, until all the oil is completely emulsified. This process can take up to 1 minute.
4. When creamy and the oil is completely emulsified, remove the blender.
5. Serve immediately or cap the jar and refrigerate for up to 1 week.

HIGH-SPEED BLENDER VERSION

1. Add the egg, mustard, salt, and lemon juice to the blender.
2. With the blender on medium speed, slowly add the olive oil through the hole in the lid and blend until the oil has emulsified and the mixture is thick and creamy, 30 to 60 seconds.

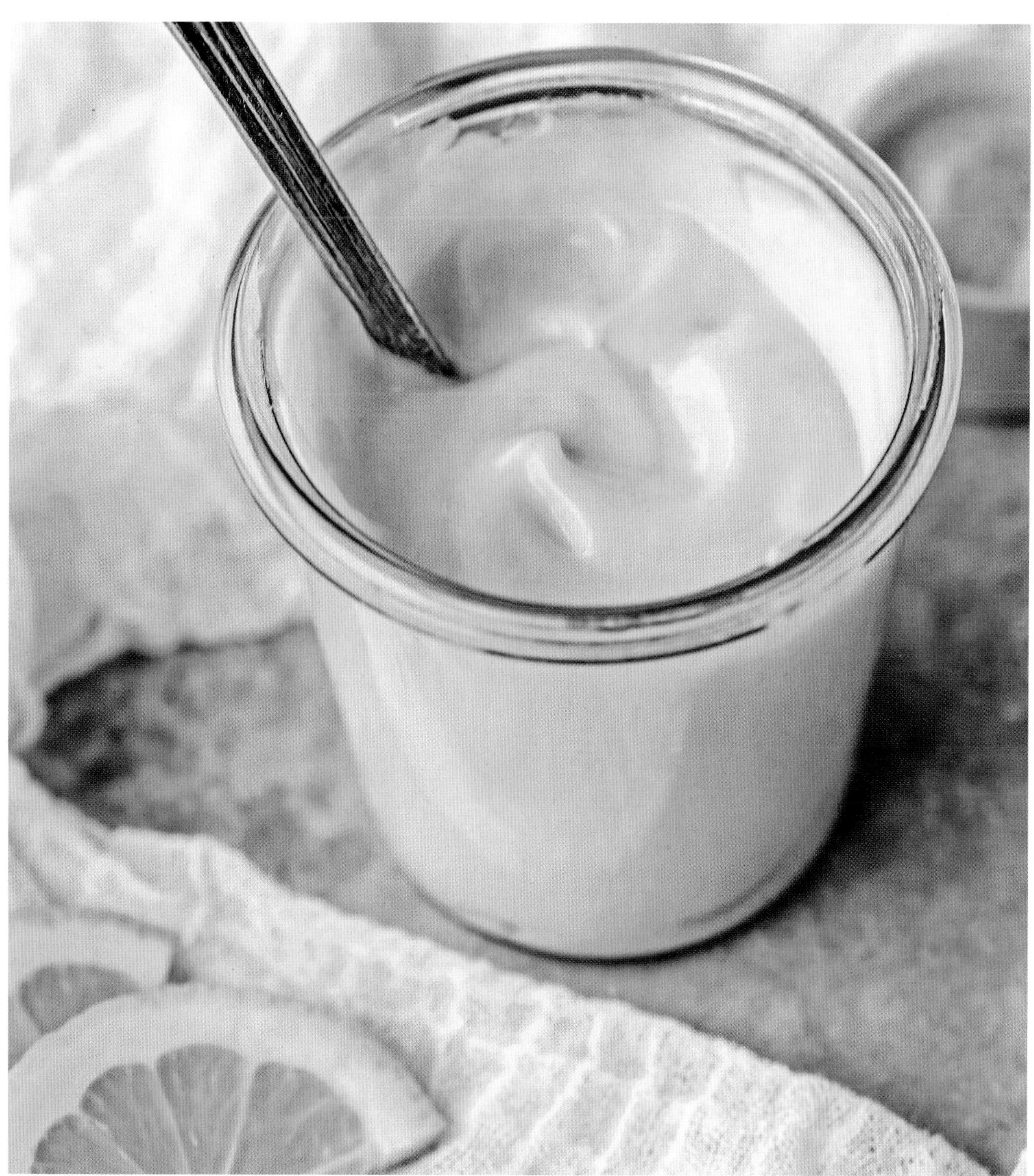

Ranch Dressing

Ranch dressing typically contains buttermilk, but this Paleo version is so good, you'll never believe it's dairy free.

SQUEAKY CLEAN PALEO / KETO PALEO / TRADITIONAL PALEO

Makes: 1 to 1¼ cups (240 to 300 ml) / **Prep Time:** 2 minutes / **Total Time:** 5 minutes

- 1 cup (240 g) Mayo (page 28) or compliant mayonnaise
- Sea salt, to taste
- 1 tablespoon (2 g) dried parsley
- 1 tablespoon (2 g) dried chives
- 2 teaspoons dried dill weed
- ½ teaspoon garlic powder
- ½ teaspoon onion powder
- ½ teaspoon cracked black pepper
- 2 tablespoons (30 ml) canned unsweetened coconut milk
- 1 teaspoon apple cider vinegar
- 1 teaspoon white wine vinegar

1. Add the mayo to a wide-mouth mason jar or medium bowl.
2. Add the salt, parsley, chives, dill, garlic powder, onion powder, and pepper to the mayo and mix together with a spoon or blend with an immersion blender for a smoother consistency (may also use a regular blender).
3. Add the coconut milk and vinegars to the seasoned mayo. Add less or more coconut milk, depending on the consistency you would like.
4. Stir with a spoon until combined. Taste and add up to 1 teaspoon more dill, if desired.
5. Cap the jar and store in the fridge for up to 1 week.

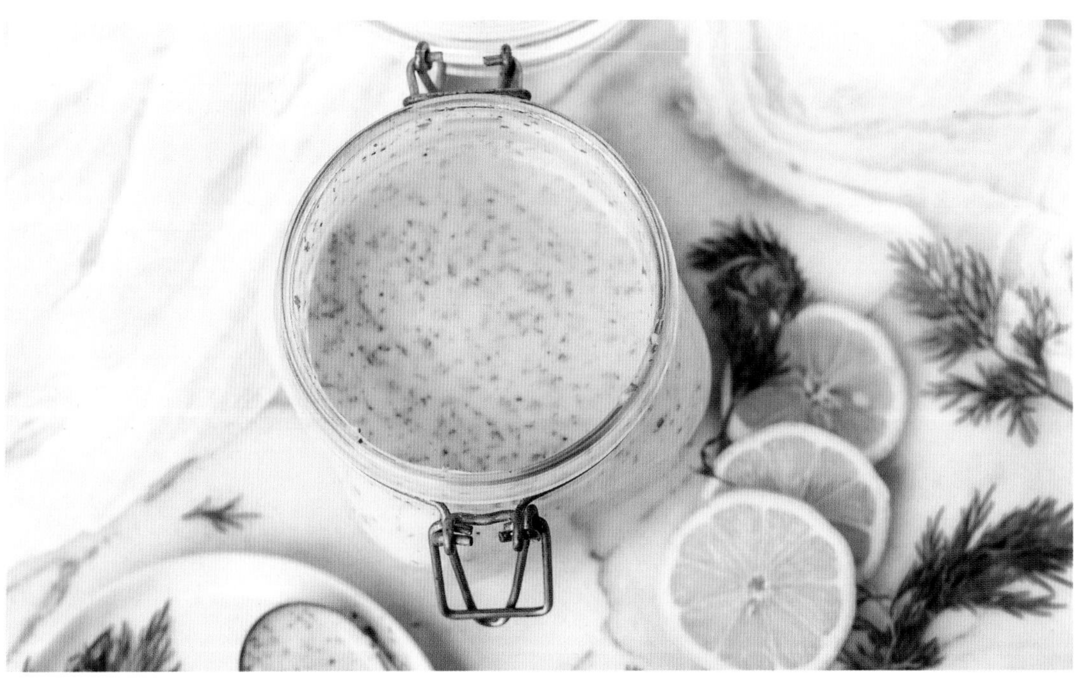

Mac's Awesome Sauce

This is my most beloved recipe on my blog, Healthy Little Peach. It's a super-simple (yet flavorful) mayo-based sauce that's infused with diced onion, coconut aminos, and black pepper. It's great on eggs, stir-fries, and roasted veggies.

SQUEAKY CLEAN PALEO / KETO PALEO / TRADITIONAL PALEO

Makes: 1 cup (240 ml) / **Prep Time:** 2 minutes / **Total Time:** 5 minutes

1 cup (240 g) Mayo (page 28) or compliant mayonnaise
1 tablespoon (10 g) chopped yellow onion
2 teaspoons coconut aminos
¾ teaspoon black pepper
Sea salt, to taste

1. Place the mayo in a wide-mouth mason jar or medium bowl.
2. Add the onion, coconut aminos, pepper, and salt.
3. Stir with a spoon until combined. Taste it and add more salt, if needed.
4. Cap the jar and refrigerate for up to 1 week.

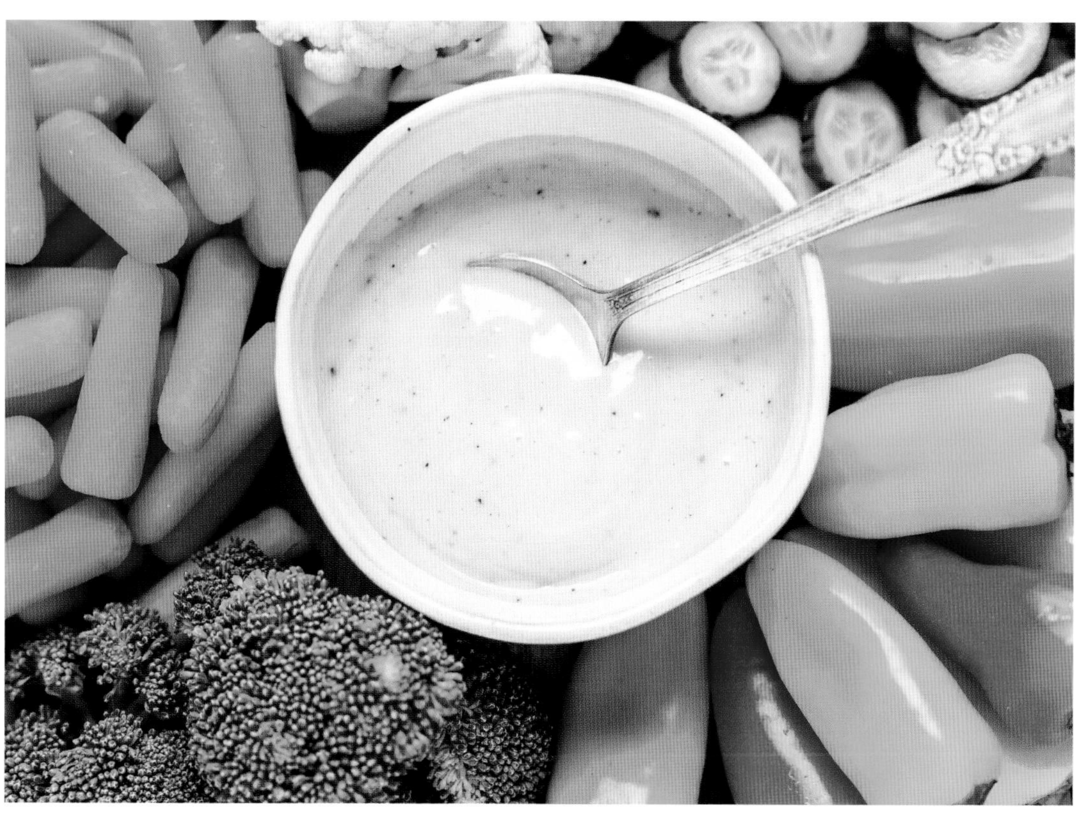

Chili Lime Sauce

This is one of those sauces that should be in your fridge on a weekly basis. It adds so much flavor to veggies, stir-fries, eggs, and bland proteins.

SQUEAKY CLEAN PALEO / KETO PALEO / TRADITIONAL PALEO

Makes: 1 cup (240 ml) / **Prep Time:** 2 minutes / **Total Time:** 5 minutes

1 cup (240 g) Mayo (page 28) or compliant mayonnaise
1 teaspoon chili powder
¼ teaspoon black pepper, or to taste
1 teaspoon lime juice
½ teaspoon lime zest
Sea salt, to taste

1. Place the mayo in a wide-mouth mason jar or medium bowl.
2. Add the chili powder, pepper, lime juice and zest, and salt.
3. Stir with a spoon until combined. Taste and add up to ½ teaspoon more salt, if needed.

Sriracha Sauce

This homemade sriracha can be whipped up in less than 20 minutes and is perfect if you are needing a little extra spice to your meals and even great to include in your Asian Paleo cooking.

SQUEAKY CLEAN PALEO / KETO PALEO / TRADITIONAL PALEO

Makes: 1½ to 1 ¾ cups (360 to 420 ml) / **Prep Time:** 10 minutes / **Total Time:** 20 minutes

¾ pound (336 g) fresh red jalapeño peppers, seeded
½ pound (224 g) fresh red mini sweet peppers, seeded
¼ cup (60 ml) apple cider vinegar
3 cloves garlic
1 tablespoon (15 g) tomato paste
2 teaspoons coconut aminos
1 teaspoon fish sauce
Sea salt, to taste

1. Add the jalapeños, red peppers, vinegar, garlic, tomato paste, coconut aminos, fish sauce, and salt to a blender or food processor. Blend until smooth, 30 to 40 seconds. If needed, add water to get consistency you want. Taste and add more salt if necessary.
2. Pour the sauce into a small saucepan. Heat over low heat to allow the flavors to come together, 10 minutes. Do not bring to a boil; just warm it.
3. Remove from the heat and allow to cool completely.
4. Transfer to a mason jar, cap it, and refrigerate. Sauce will keep for 2 to 3 weeks.

Bang Bang Sauce

This spicy, Asian-inspired sauce packs a flavor punch with homemade sriracha, coconut aminos, and garlic. It's perfect on chicken, such as the Hibachi Chicken Skewers on page 115, or shrimp, such as the Shrimp Fried Rice on page 106.

SQUEAKY CLEAN PALEO / KETO PALEO / TRADITIONAL PALEO

Makes: ½ to ¾ cup (120 to 180 ml) / **Prep Time:** 2 minutes / **Total Time:** 7 minutes

½ cup (120 ml) Mayo (page 28) or compliant mayonnaise

2½ tablespoons (37 ml) Sriracha Sauce (page 32) or no-sugar-added sriracha sauce

1 teaspoon coconut aminos

½ teaspoon garlic powder

1. Add the mayo to a small bowl with the sriracha sauce, coconut aminos, and garlic powder.
2. Mix together with a spoon until combined.
3. Serve immediately or store in the fridge in an airtight jar for up to 1 week.

Southwest Sauce

This tangy, spicy sauce is great on pretty much anything, but especially eggs and the Steak Kabobs on page 123. Chipotle paste can be found in many international sections in most grocery stores or online.

SQUEAKY CLEAN PALEO / KETO PALEO / TRADITIONAL PALEO

Makes: 1 to 1¼ cups (240 to 300 ml) / **Prep Time:** 5 minutes / **Total Time:** 8 minutes

1 cup (240 g) Mayo (page 28) or compliant mayonnaise
1 tablespoon (12 g) chipotle paste
½ teaspoon garlic powder
Sea salt, to taste
¼ teaspoon onion powder
¼ teaspoon ground cumin
2 tablespoons (2 g) coarsely chopped cilantro
Juice of ½ lime

1. Add the mayo and chipotle paste to a wide-mouth mason jar or medium bowl.
2. Add the garlic powder, salt, onion powder, cumin, cilantro, and lime juice.
3. Use an immersion blender to combine all ingredients well. Cap the jar and refrigerate for up to 1 week.

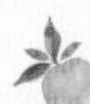

RECIPE NOTES

If you don't have an immersion blender, put all the ingredients into a blender and blend on high until combined. If you can't find chipotle paste, substitute 3 chiles in compliant adobe sauce.

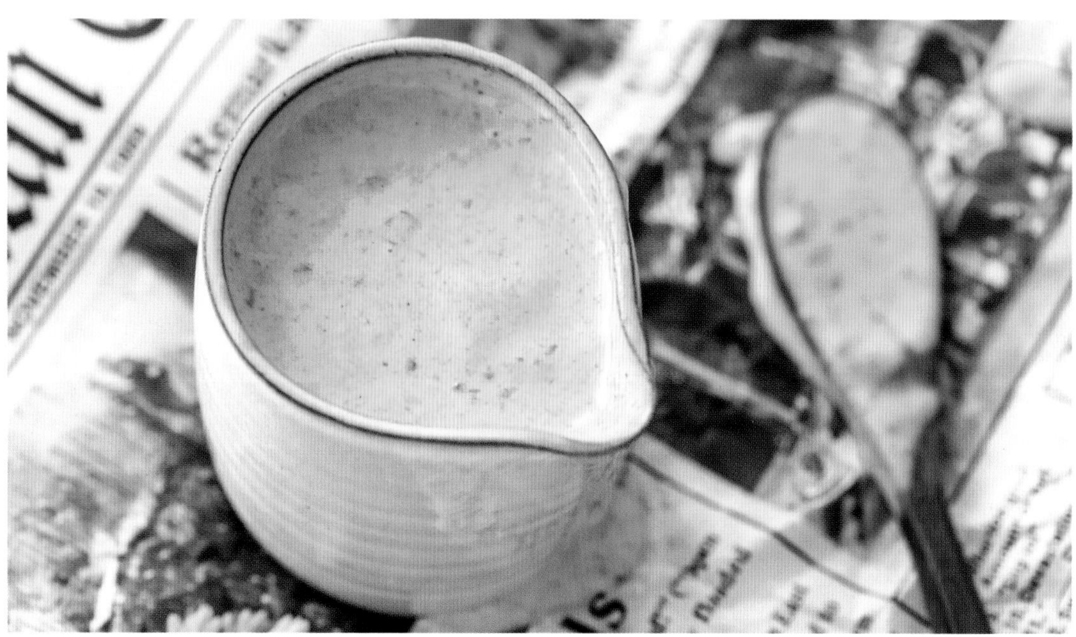

BBQ Sauce

Store-bought BBQ sauce typically packs in the unpronounceable ingredients. And homemade versions amp up the brown sugar and ketchup and can take an hour to make. This Paleo version uses dates for sweetness and is both simple and quick to make. Add it to shredded pork (such as the one in chapter 7), chicken, or pork chops to add tons of flavor. You can even use it as a dipping sauce for Paleo chicken tenders.

SQUEAKY CLEAN PALEO / KETO PALEO / TRADITIONAL PALEO

Makes: 1 cup (240 ml) / **Prep Time:** 5 minutes / **Total Time:** 10 minutes

- 1 can (8 ounces [224 g]) no-sugar-added tomato sauce
- 1 can (6 ounces [168 g]) tomato paste
- ⅓ cup (80 ml) coconut aminos
- ¼ cup (60 ml) balsamic vinegar
- 7 Medjool dates, pitted or 2½ tablespoons of monk fruit syrup if Keto
- 2 tablespoons (30 ml) apple cider vinegar
- 1½ tablespoons (9 g) chili powder
- 1 tablespoon (11 g) no sugar added Dijon mustard
- 2 teaspoons paprika
- 1 teaspoon onion powder
- Sea salt, to taste
- 1 teaspoon black pepper

1. To a blender, add the tomato sauce, tomato paste, coconut aminos, balsamic vinegar, dates, apple cider vinegar, chili powder, mustard, paprika, onion powder, salt, and pepper. Blend on high speed until smooth, about 30 seconds.
2. Pour into a small saucepan and heat over low until warm (not boiling), about 4 minutes. Remove from the heat and let cool.
3. Transfer the sauce to a mason jar, cap it, and store in the fridge for up to 4 weeks.

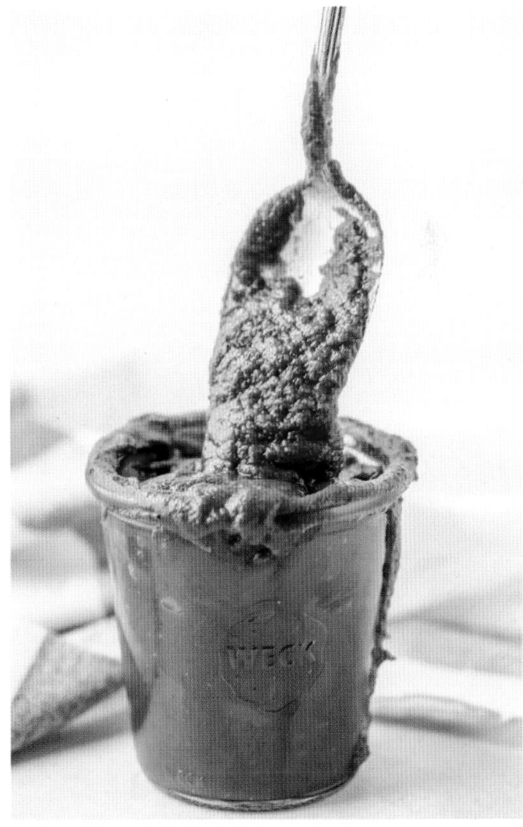

Peach Vinaigrette

If you look at the labels on store-bought vinaigrettes, you'll often find sugar as one of the first ingredients; some brands even use corn syrup! This delicious vinaigrette is sweetened with peach to make the best sweet-savory dressing. Use it on salads, chicken, or pork, such as the Grilled Pork Chops with Peach Vinaigrette on page 105.

SQUEAKY CLEAN PALEO / TRADITIONAL PALEO

Makes: ½ cup to ¾ cup (120 to 180 ml) / **Prep Time:** 5 minutes / **Total Time:** 10 minutes

---

1 large peach, peeled and pitted
¼ cup (60 ml) light olive oil
¼ cup (60 ml) white wine vinegar
1 tablespoon (15 ml) lemon juice
1 tablespoon (11 g) Dijon mustard
1 tablespoon (15 ml) coconut aminos
2 cloves garlic
Sea salt, to taste
1 teaspoon black pepper

---

1. Add the peach, olive oil, vinegar, lemon juice, mustard, coconut aminos, garlic, salt, and pepper to a blender or food processor.
2. Blend on medium to high speed until creamy, 30 to 40 seconds.
3. Transfer to a jar, cap it, and refrigerate for up to 1 week.

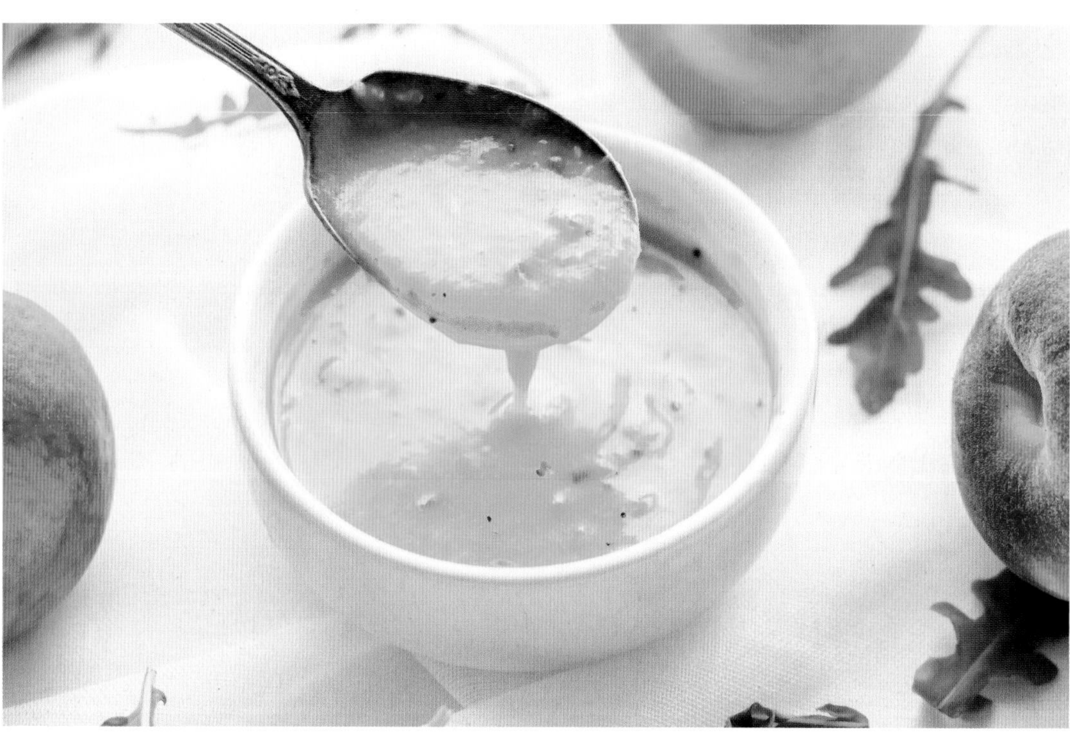

Greek Dressing

Who doesn't enjoy a traditional Greek salad, especially that tangy dressing? This Paleo version hits all the notes and is ridiculously easy to make.

SQUEAKY CLEAN PALEO / KETO PALEO / TRADITIONAL PALEO

Makes: ¾ cup (180 ml) / **Prep Time:** 2 minutes / **Total Time:** 5 minutes

½ cup (120 ml) light olive oil
¼ cup (60 ml) red wine vinegar
2 tablespoons (30 ml) lemon juice
2 cloves garlic, minced
1¼ teaspoons Dijon mustard
1 teaspoon dried oregano
½ teaspoon dried basil
Sea salt, to taste
¼ teaspoon cracked black pepper, plus more to taste

1. Add the olive oil, vinegar, lemon juice, garlic, mustard, oregano, basil, salt, and pepper to a blender or food processor.
2. Blend on medium to high speed until creamy, 15 to 30 seconds. Taste and add more pepper, if desired.
3. Transfer to a jar, cap it, and refrigerate for up to 1 week.

Basil Pesto

Traditional pesto sauce relies on Parmesan or pecorino cheese. Here, I've swapped the non-Paleo ingredient with cheesy-tasting nutritional yeast. It's simple yet flavorful, and it can bring any protein or veggie to life. Try it on veggie spirals!

SQUEAKY CLEAN PALEO / KETO PALEO / TRADITIONAL PALEO

Makes: 1 to 1½ cups (240 to 360 g) / **Prep Time:** 5 minutes / **Total Time:** 10 minutes

2 cups (80 g) fresh basil leaves
1 cup (30 g) baby spinach
⅓ cup (45 g) pine nuts
1 clove garlic, coarsely chopped
3 tablespoons (45 ml) lemon juice
2 tablespoons (4 g) nutritional yeast
1 teaspoon lemon zest
Sea salt and black pepper, to taste
½ cup (120 ml) light olive oil

1. Rinse the basil and spinach and pat dry with a paper towel. Set aside.
2. Add the pine nuts and garlic to a food processor and process until smooth, about 20 seconds.
3. Add the basil, spinach, lemon juice, nutritional yeast, lemon zest, salt, and pepper. Pulse 4 to 5 times to break up the leaves.
4. Turn the food processor on low and slowly add the olive oil through the feed tube until everything is well combined.
5. Serve immediately or store in an airtight container in the fridge for up to 4 days.

Avocado Cilantro Cream

Don't let the name fool you. This avocado cream has no dairy and is infused with lime juice and cilantro. It pairs nicely with tacos (such as Crispy Fish Tacos on page 134), fajitas (such as Sheet Pan Steak Fajitas on page 103), or even just plain old chicken.

SQUEAKY CLEAN PALEO / KETO PALEO / TRADITIONAL PALEO

Makes: 1 cup (240 ml) / **Prep Time:** 5 minutes / **Total Time:** 10 minutes

1 avocado, peeled and pitted
2 handfuls cilantro (about 2 cups [32 g])
⅓ cup (80 ml) light olive oil
Juice of 1 lime
2 cloves garlic
1 teaspoon paprika
½ teaspoon sea salt
¼ teaspoon black pepper
¼ teaspoon onion powder

1. Add the avocado, cilantro, olive oil, lime juice, garlic, paprika, salt, pepper, and onion powder to a blender or food processor.
2. Blend on high speed until creamy, 30 to 40 seconds.
3. Serve immediately or store, covered, in the fridge overnight. It's best used within 1 day as the avocado may turn brown.

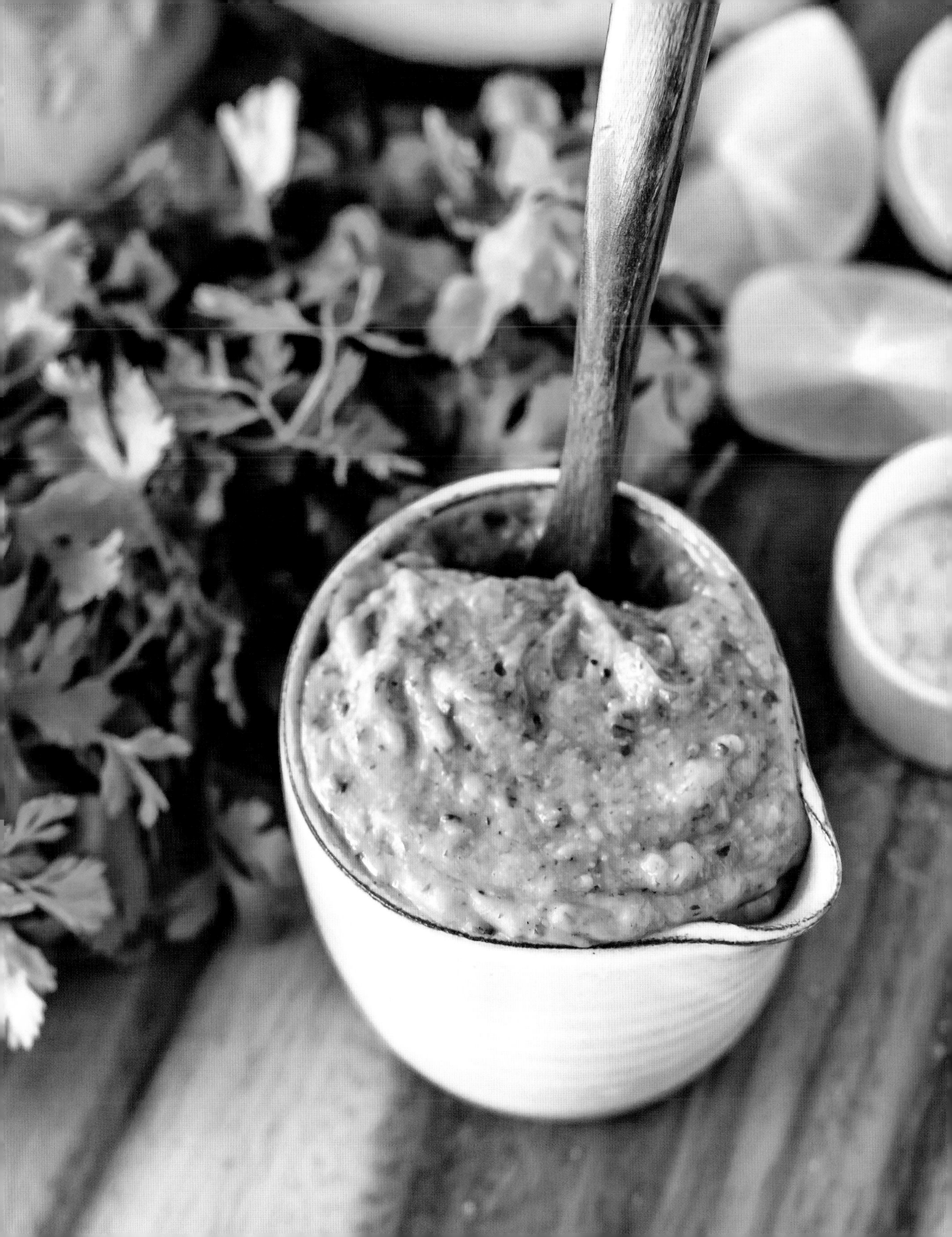

Cashew Queso

This creamy, dairy-free alternative tastes identical to the real thing. And it's just as versatile. Drizzle it on nachos, or dip in with plantain chips or sweet potato fries. Layering cashew cream, seasoned ground beef, tomatoes, and scallions makes for the perfect queso dip.

SQUEAKY CLEAN PALEO / KETO PALEO / TRADITIONAL PALEO

Makes: 6 servings / **Prep Time:** 2 minutes / **Total Time:** 5 minutes + cashew soaking time

1¼ cups (180 g) raw unsalted cashews, soaked in water for at least 3 hours, drained, and rinsed
1 cup (240 ml) hot water
¼ cup (16 g) nutritional yeast
3 tablespoons (45 ml) compliant, no sugar added chicken broth
2 tablespoons (30 ml) lemon juice
½ teaspoon garlic powder
½ teaspoon sea salt
½ teaspoon chili powder

1. Add the cashews, hot water, nutritional yeast, broth, lemon juice, garlic powder, salt, and chili powder to a high-speed blender or food processor and blend until creamy and smooth, 60 seconds. If it gets too thin, thicken with additional raw cashews, and if it is too thick, add additional water to get the perfect texture.
2. Store leftovers, covered, in the refrigerator for 5 to 7 days.

RECIPE NOTES

For serving, try topping the queso with ½ cup (100 g) cooked ground beef, 2 tablespoons (23 g) diced tomatoes, and 1 tablespoon (10 g) diced onion. Garnish with chopped green onions and lime.

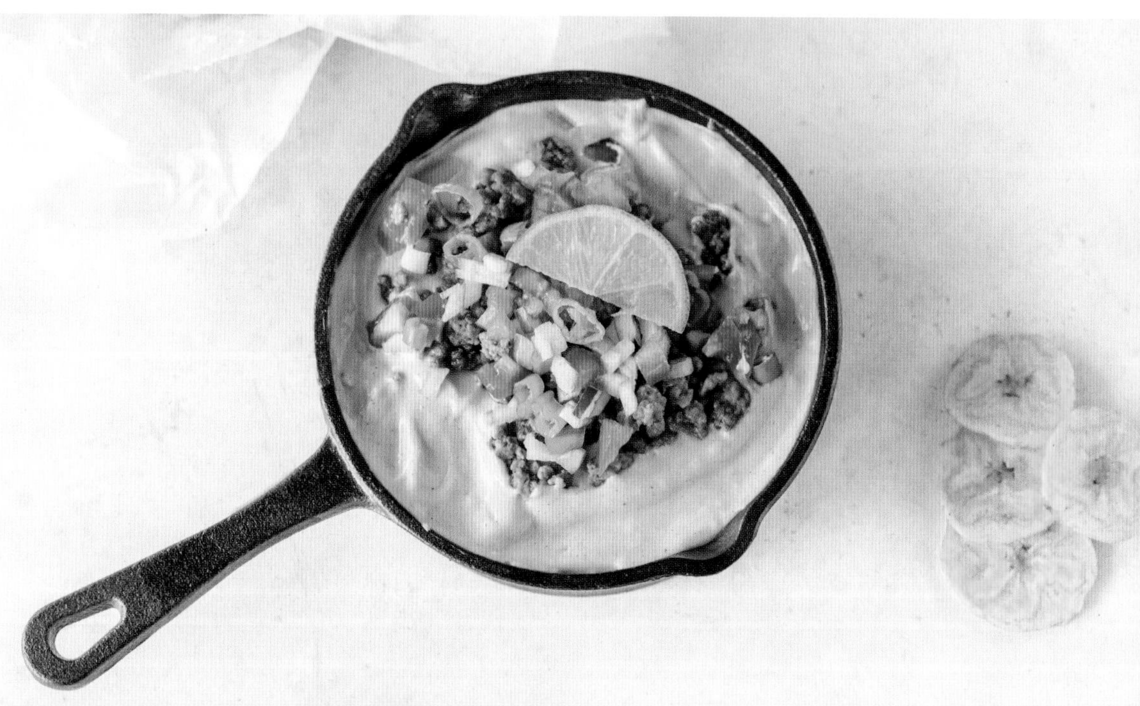

Chicken Marinade, 3 Ways

These three go-to marinades add tons of flavor to boring chicken—or even pork. They're so simple to make that you could have your chicken marinating before you leave for work and have it tender and tasty by the time you get home.

SQUEAKY CLEAN PALEO / KETO PALEO / TRADITIONAL PALEO

Makes: Enough marinade for 2 pounds (910 g) of chicken / **Prep Time:** 1 to 2 minutes / **Total Time:** 5 minutes

---

CILANTRO-LIME MARINADE

2 handfuls cilantro
½ cup (120 ml) olive oil
Juice of 1 lime
2 cloves garlic, minced
1 teaspoon sea salt
½ teaspoon black pepper
¼ teaspoon onion powder

EVERYTHING MARINADE

⅓ cup (80 ml) olive oil
¼ cup (60 ml) coconut aminos
Juice of 1 lemon
2 cloves garlic, minced
2 teaspoons dried parsley

GREEK MARINADE

½ cup (120 ml) olive oil
Juice of 1 large lemon
1 tablespoon (15 ml) red wine vinegar
1 tablespoon (2 g) dried oregano
2 cloves garlic, minced
1 teaspoon sea salt
½ teaspoon dried basil
½ teaspoon cracked black pepper

TO USE

1. Add all the ingredients for each marinade to a food processor or blender and process until completely combined.
2. Transfer the marinade to a 1-gallon (3.6 L) resealable plastic bag and add the chicken. Seal and gently toss to coat all the chicken with the marinade. Set in a dish or pan and refrigerate. For maximum flavor, marinate for 6 to 12 hours, or overnight.

Asian Meatballs

Who needs takeout when you can make these delicious meatballs with a sticky Asian sauce? It might take a little bit longer to make than it would to call in an order, but you'll have the satisfaction of knowing that there are no unhealthy ingredients here! Serve them with cauliflower rice and green beans to get the full takeout effect.

SQUEAKY CLEAN PALEO / KETO PALEO / TRADITIONAL PALEO

Makes: 18 to 20 meatballs / **Prep Time:** 5 minutes / **Total Time:** 35 minutes

MEATBALLS

- 2 pounds (910 g) 90/10 ground beef
- ½ cup (48 g) almond flour
- ⅓ cup (53 g) chopped onion
- 1 large egg
- 1 tablespoon (15 ml) coconut aminos
- ½ teaspoon ground ginger
- ½ teaspoon ground garlic
- ½ teaspoon sea salt
- ½ teaspoon black pepper
- 2 large scallions, chopped, for garnish
- Sesame seeds, for garnish

ASIAN STICKY SAUCE

- 1 cup (240 ml) coconut aminos
- ½ cup (120 ml) rice vinegar
- 1½ teaspoons sesame oil
- 1 clove garlic, minced
- ½ teaspoon ground ginger
- 1 tablespoon (6 g) arrowroot powder, dissolved in 1½ tablespoons (23 ml) water (see Note for Keto)

MEATBALLS

1. Preheat the oven to 400°F (200°C or gas mark 6) and coat a baking sheet with olive oil or cooking spray.
2. Add the ground beef, almond flour, onion, egg, coconut aminos, ginger, garlic, salt, and pepper to a large bowl. Mix together with your hands until well combined. (Add a little more almond flour if the mixture is still too wet.)
3. Form the meatball mixture into golf ball–size balls; you should have 18 to 20. Place them on the prepared baking sheet.
4. Bake until the meatballs are browned and reach an internal temperature of 160°F (71°C), 20 to 25 minutes.

ASIAN STICKY SAUCE

1. Place the coconut aminos, vinegar, sesame oil, garlic, and ginger in a small saucepan and set over medium-high heat.
2. Once the mixture is hot, add the dissolved arrowroot mixture. Reduce the heat to low and stir frequently. As the sauce heats, it will begin to thicken. This may take a few minutes.
3. Spoon the meatballs along with the sauce onto a plate. Serve sprinkled with the scallions and sesame seeds.

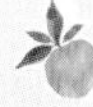

RECIPE NOTES

You can substitute tapioca flour for arrowroot. If you're Keto, use ¼ teaspoon xanthan gum or 1½ tablespoons (14 g) gelatin.

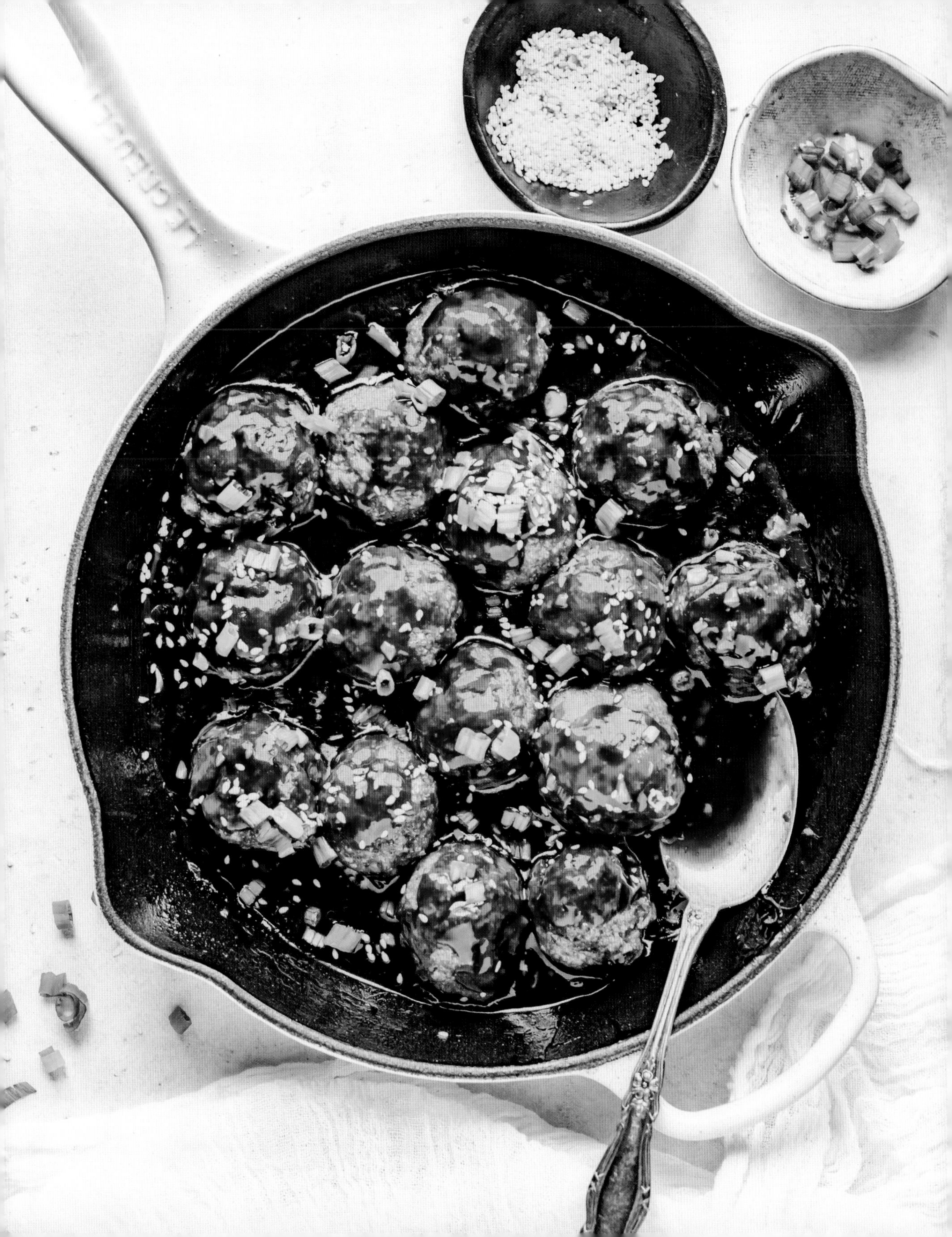
LE CREUSET

Buffalo, Dill, and Bacon Wings

These traditional chicken wings get an extra flavor bump when they're tossed in a creamy dill-infused buffalo sauce. Then I up the ante by topping them with crispy bacon. You almost won't want to share them!

SQUEAKY CLEAN PALEO / KETO PALEO / TRADITIONAL PALEO

Makes: Approximately 20 wings + 1 cup (240 ml) sauce / **Prep Time:** 10 minutes / **Total Time:** 40 minutes

BUFFALO DILL SAUCE

1 cup (240 g) Mayo (page 28) or compliant mayonnaise
2 teaspoons compliant hot sauce
1½ teaspoons dried dill weed
1 teaspoon black pepper
Sea salt, to taste

CHICKEN WINGS

2 pounds (910 g) chicken wings
2 tablespoons (30 ml) olive oil
Sea salt and black pepper, to taste
⅓ cup (80 ml) Buffalo Dill Sauce
4 slices cooked compliant bacon, crumbled (see Tip)
Fresh dill, for garnish

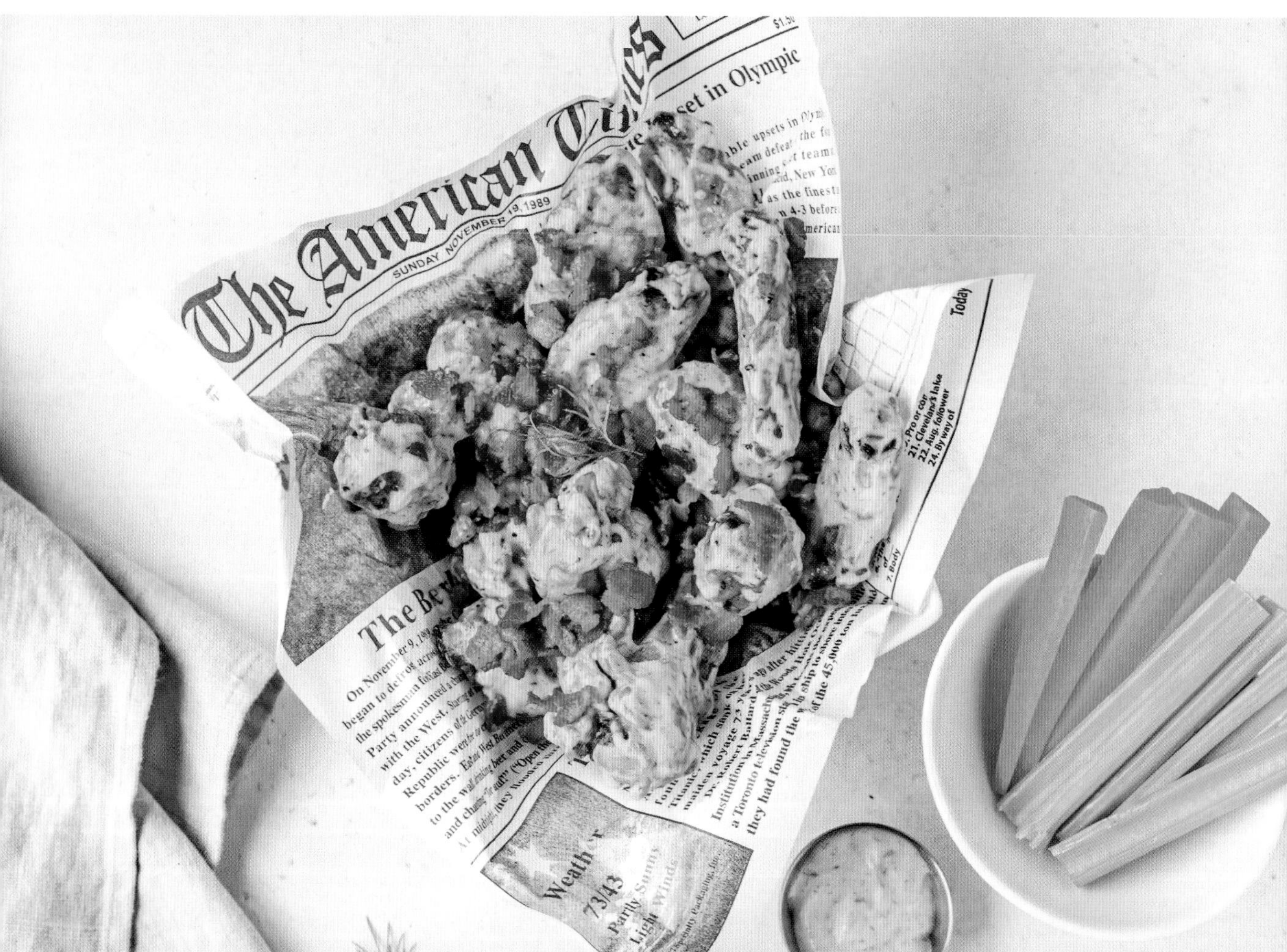

BUFFALO DILL SAUCE

1. Place the mayo in a wide-mouth mason jar or medium bowl.
2. Add the hot sauce, dill, pepper, and salt.
3. Stir with a spoon until combined. Taste and add up to ½ teaspoon more salt, if needed.
4. Cap the jar and refrigerate for up to 1 week.

OVEN METHOD

1. Preheat the oven to 425°F (220°C or gas mark 7) and coat a baking sheet with olive oil cooking spray.
2. Pat the wings dry with a paper towel. Place them in a bowl and drizzle with the olive oil, turning until each wing is coated.
3. Place the wings on the prepared baking sheet with space between each wing. Sprinkle them with salt and pepper.
4. Bake for 15 minutes, then remove the wings from the oven and turn them. Return to the oven and bake until the outside is golden and crispy and the internal temperature reads 160°F (71°C), 15 to 20 minutes more.
5. Transfer the wings to a large mixing bowl. Pour the Buffalo Dill Sauce over them and mix until each wing is covered. Serve garnished with the bacon crumbles and fresh dill.

AIR FRYER METHOD

1. Prep the air fryer basket by spraying with olive oil cooking spray and turning to 380°F (192°C).
2. Pat the wings dry with a paper towel. Place them in a bowl and drizzle with the olive oil, turning until each wing is coated. Sprinkle the wings with salt and pepper.
3. Add the wings to the basket and cook for 25 minutes. Make sure to shake the basket every 5 minutes to ensure even cooking. After 25 minutes, shake the wings one more time. Increase the temperature to 400°F (200°C) and cook for 5 minutes more.
4. Remove the basket and transfer the wings to a large mixing bowl. Pour the Buffalo Dill Sauce over them and mix until each wing is covered. Serve garnished with the bacon crumbles and fresh dill.

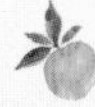

TIP

Perfectly cook bacon on a baking sheet in a 400°F (200°C or gas mark 6) oven for 15 to 20 minutes, or until desired doneness. Transfer to a paper towel to drain, and then chop on a cutting board.

RECIPE NOTES

Add more or less of the Buffalo Dill Sauce, depending on how coated you like your wings.

Chive and Onion Mixed Nuts

These mixed nuts are the perfect snack or salad-topping option. They taste identical to a sour cream and onion potato chip—but without all the bad stuff.

SQUEAKY CLEAN PALEO / KETO PALEO / TRADITIONAL PALEO

Makes: 3½ cups (508 g) / **Prep Time:** 3 minutes / **Total Time:** 13 minutes

3½ cups (508 g) unsalted mixed nuts (pecans, cashews, pistachios, almonds, and hazelnuts)
1½ tablespoons (23 ml) olive oil
1 tablespoon (2 g) dried chives
2 teaspoons onion powder
1 teaspoon garlic powder
1 teaspoon sea salt

1. Preheat the oven to 350°F (180°C or gas mark 4). Line a baking sheet with parchment paper.
2. In a large mixing bowl, combine the nuts with the olive oil, chives, onion powder, garlic powder, and salt. Mix together until the nuts are evenly coated.
3. Spread the nuts on the prepared baking sheet.
4. Bake until golden brown, about 10 to 13 minutes. Remove from the oven and allow the nuts to cool before serving. If desired, sprinkle a pinch of salt over all the nuts right when they come out of the oven.
5. Store in an airtight container for up to 2 weeks.

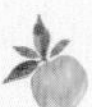

RECIPE NOTES

Keep an eye on the nuts as they bake to make sure they don't burn. All ovens are different, so adjust the bake time as needed.

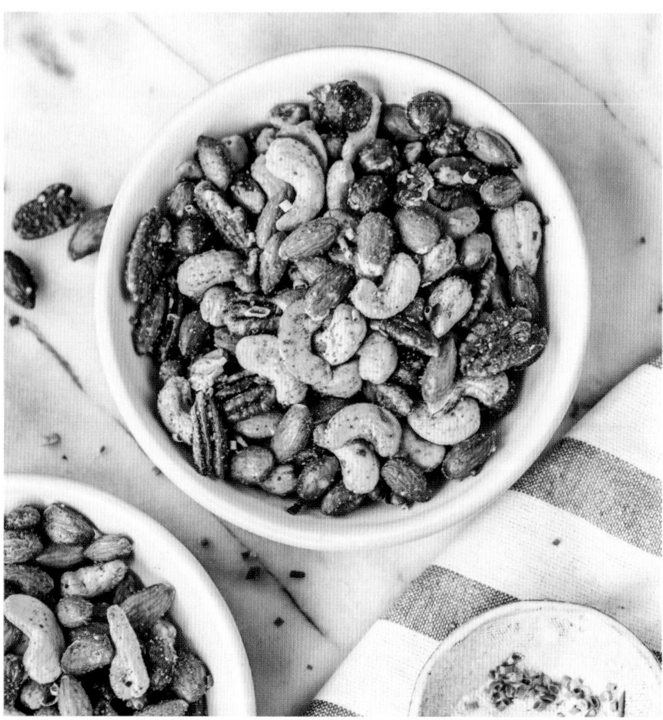

Tostones and Shredded Pork Nachos

Tostones are twice-fried plantain slices. Because they become so crispy, I thought they'd make the perfect base for nachos! Here, I top them with Shredded Pork (page 142), red onion, tomatoes, cilantro, and Cashew Queso (page 40) to make them Paleo friendly.

SQUEAKY CLEAN PALEO / TRADITIONAL PALEO

Makes: 4 servings / **Prep Time:** 10 minutes / **Total Time:** 25 minutes

- 1 cup (240 g) coconut oil, divided
- 3 large green plantains, peeled and cut into 1-inch (2.5 cm) chunks
- 1 teaspoon sea salt
- 1½ pounds (680 g) prepared Shredded Pork (see Note on page 142)
- ¼ cup (40 g) diced red onion
- ¼ cup (36 g) sliced jalapeño
- ⅓ cup (50 g) diced Roma tomatoes
- 2 tablespoons (30 g) compliant salsa
- Fresh chopped cilantro, for garnish
- Optional: Cashew Queso (page 40) or Ranch Dressing (page 30)

1. Heat ½ cup (120 g) of the coconut oil in a large skillet over medium-high heat. Place the plantains in the oil and fry until browned on both sides, 3 to 4 minutes per side.
2. Remove the plantains from the skillet, placing them one at a time in between two pieces of parchment paper. Use a flat surface, such as the bottom of a glass, to press down and flatten the plantain. Set aside until they're all flattened.
3. Add the remaining ½ cup (120 g) coconut oil to the skillet. When hot, return the flattened plantains to the skillet and fry until golden and crispy, 1 minute on each side.
4. Remove the crispy tostones to a baking sheet and sprinkle with the salt.
5. Now begin to build the nachos in this order: tostones, shredded pork, onion, jalapeño, tomatoes, salsa, and cilantro.
6. Serve immediately, drizzled with Cashew Queso or Ranch Dressing, if desired.

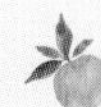

RECIPE NOTES

This is a great recipe to make if you have leftover shredded pork from a previous dinner. If not, luckily the pork is a snap to make in the slow cooker if you set it before you leave for work in the morning, or the electric pressure cooker, if you need to make it when you come home. You can also find premade compliant shredded pork at some grocery stores.

Buffalo Chicken Patties with Southwest Ranch

This recipe is in honor of my husband, Joel, who is constantly begging for a buffalo recipe that is unique, healthy, *and* delicious. These slightly spicy patties will please any guy, woman, or kid in the house.

SQUEAKY CLEAN PALEO / KETO PALEO / TRADITIONAL PALEO

Makes: 8 patties and about 1 cup (240 ml) sauce / **Prep Time:** 5 minutes / **Total Time:** 25 minutes

BUFFALO CHICKEN PATTIES

2 pounds (910 g) ground chicken
½ sweet onion, diced
1 large egg, beaten
⅓ cup (32 g) almond flour
3 tablespoons (45 ml) compliant hot sauce
1 teaspoon garlic powder
1 teaspoon sea salt
1 teaspoon black pepper
1 teaspoon compliant mayo
2 tablespoons (28 g) ghee, divided
¼ cup (25 g) sliced scallion

SOUTHWEST RANCH

1 cup (240 ml) Ranch Dressing (page 30)
2 tablespoons (30 ml) compliant hot sauce
1 teaspoon lime juice

BUFFALO CHICKEN PATTIES

1. In a large mixing bowl, place the chicken, onion, egg, flour, hot sauce, garlic powder, salt, pepper, and mayo. Mix together using your hands until everything is combined.
2. Divide the mixture into 8 portions and use your hands to roll each into balls. Add more almond flour as needed if the mixture is too wet. Place on a plate or piece of parchment paper. (If you want to make more patties that are even cuter as tiny apps, form into smaller balls.)
3. Heat 1 tablespoon (14 g) of the ghee in a large skillet over medium-high heat until the ghee sizzles.
4. Add 4 patties to the skillet and use a spatula to press each ball into a disk shape.
5. Cook the patties until golden brown and the internal temperature reaches 160°F (71°C), 4 to 5 minutes on each side.
6. Remove the patties to a plate and cover to keep warm. Repeat with the remaining 1 tablespoon (14 g) ghee and 4 patties.
7. To serve, drizzle with the spicy ranch and sprinkle with the scallions.

SOUTHWEST RANCH

In a mason jar or medium bowl, use a spoon to combine the ranch, hot sauce, and lime juice. Cap the jar and store in the fridge for up to 1 week.

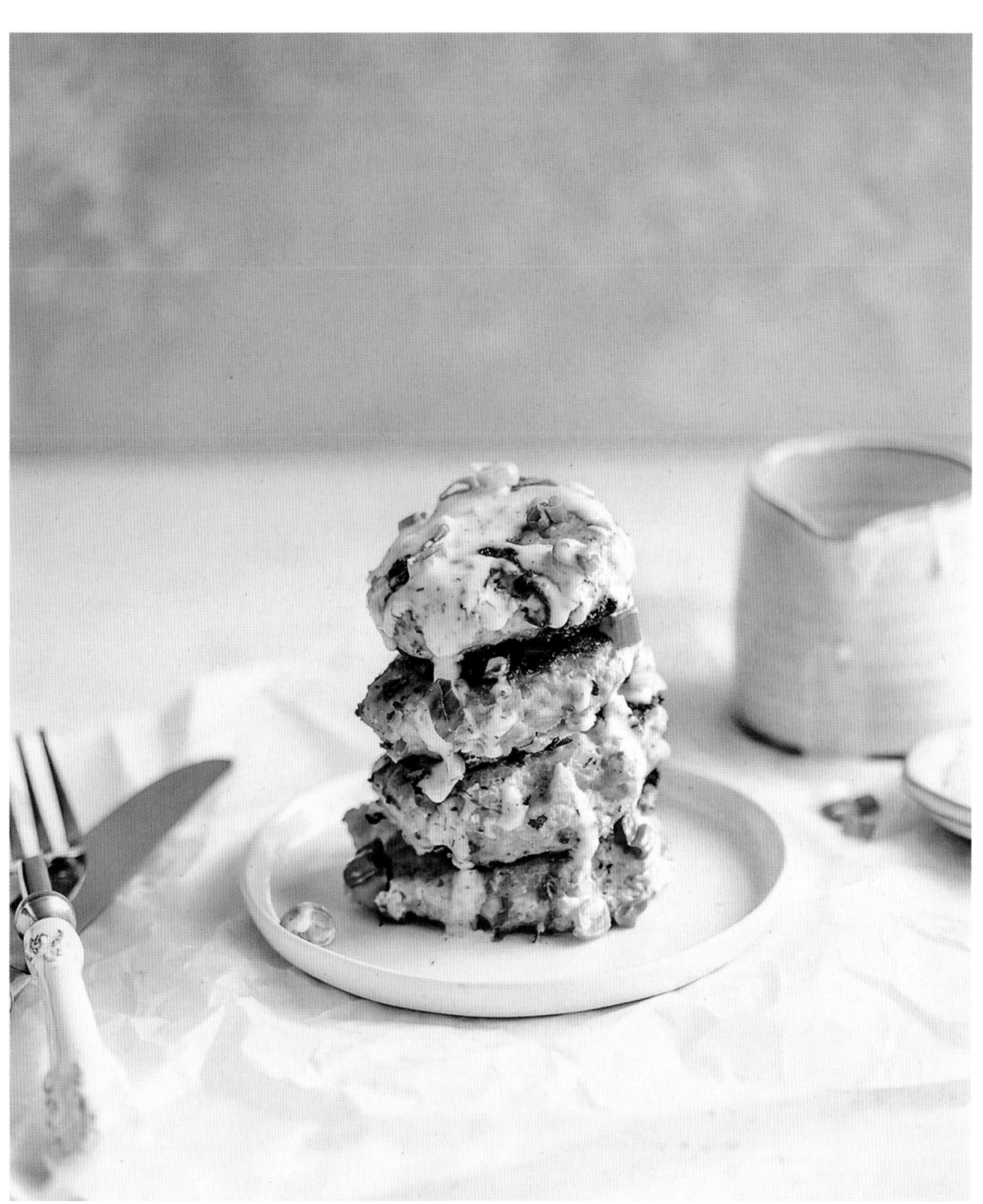

Zucchini and Onion Fritters

These fritters are a simple and delicious way to get in your veggies. It's also a great way to use up that bumper crop of zucchini come July! These will pair great with my Mac's Awesome Sauce (page 31) or Chili Lime Sauce (page 32).

SQUEAKY CLEAN PALEO / KETO PALEO / TRADITIONAL PALEO

Makes: Eleven 2½-inch (6.3 cm) fritters / **Prep Time:** 10 minutes / **Total Time:** 25 minutes

---

1½ pounds (680 g) zucchini (about 4 medium), grated
1 teaspoon sea salt, plus more for seasoning
½ yellow onion, chopped
2 large eggs
⅓ cup (32 g) almond flour
2½ tablespoons (15 g) arrowroot powder
2 tablespoons (8 g) nutritional yeast (optional)
1½ teaspoons dried chives
½ teaspoon black pepper
¼ teaspoon onion powder
2 tablespoons (28 g) ghee, divided
2 or 3 scallions, chopped, for garnish

---

1. Place the zucchini in a colander set over a bowl. Sprinkle with the salt. Set aside for 8 to 10 minutes, pressing down during this time to push as much water as possible out of the zucchini.
2. Transfer the zucchini to a paper towel or clean kitchen towel and squeeze tightly to get out more liquid.
3. In a large bowl, whisk together the onion, eggs, almond flour, arrowroot, nutritional yeast (if using), chives, pepper, and onion powder.
4. Add the zucchini and mix well.
5. Heat 1 tablespoon (14 g) of the ghee in a large skillet over medium-high heat until the ghee sizzles.
6. Working in batches, drop heaping tablespoons (15 g) of batter into the skillet. (You'll only use about half the batter.) Flatten slightly with the back of a spoon or spatula. Cook, turning once, until browned on both sides, 4 to 6 minutes each.
7. Transfer the fritters to a plate lined with a paper towel and sprinkle with sea salt. Repeat with the remaining 1 tablespoon (14 g) ghee and batter.
8. Sprinkle with the scallions before serving.

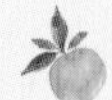

RECIPE NOTES

To make this Keto Paleo, subsitute the arrowroot flour with ½ tablespoon of coconut flour.

Chili-Lime Deviled Eggs

A spin on the traditional deviled eggs, these eggs are filled with chili-lime flavors that really bring them to life. Great for both parties and snacking.

SQUEAKY CLEAN PALEO / KETO PALEO / TRADITIONAL PALEO

Makes: 16 deviled eggs / **Prep Time:** 3 minutes / **Total Time:** 20 minutes

8 large eggs
½ cup (120 ml) Chili Lime Sauce (page 32)
1 teaspoon apple cider vinegar
1 teaspoon lime juice
½ teaspoon chili powder
½ teaspoon sea salt
½ teaspoon black pepper
Paprika, for garnish
Chopped fresh chives, for garnish

1. Place the eggs in a single layer in a saucepan and cover them with cool water. Heat over high heat until the water begins to boil, then cover with a lid and turn the heat to low. Cook for a minute or two, then remove the pan from the heat. Leave the eggs, covered, for an additional 13 minutes.
2. Meanwhile, prepare an ice bath by adding ice and water to a large bowl. Use a slotted spoon to transfer the boiled eggs to the ice water. Allow to sit for a couple of minutes, until cool enough to handle.
3. Peel the eggs and place them on a paper towel to dry.
4. Slice each egg in half lengthwise. Gently remove the yolks with a spoon, transferring them to a medium bowl. Place the whites on a platter.
5. Mash the yolks into a smooth crumble using a fork.
6. Add the Chili Lime Sauce, vinegar, lime juice, chili powder, salt, and pepper. Mix together until combined evenly.
7. Pipe the yolk mixture with a piping bag, or spoon the mixture, into each egg white half. Garnish with paprika and chives.

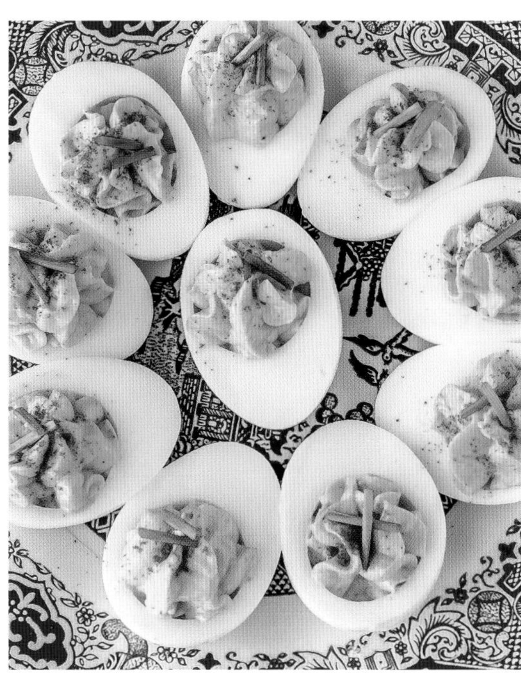

Air Fryer Pickles

Crispy air fryer pickles are perfect for when you need a little something extra. They're out-of-this-world good when dipped in the Boom Boom Fry Sauce.

SQUEAKY CLEAN PALEO / KETO PALEO / TRADITIONAL PALEO

Makes: 2 cups (400 g) pickle slices and about 1¼ cups (300 ml) sauce / **Prep Time:** 10 minutes

Total Time: 20 minutes

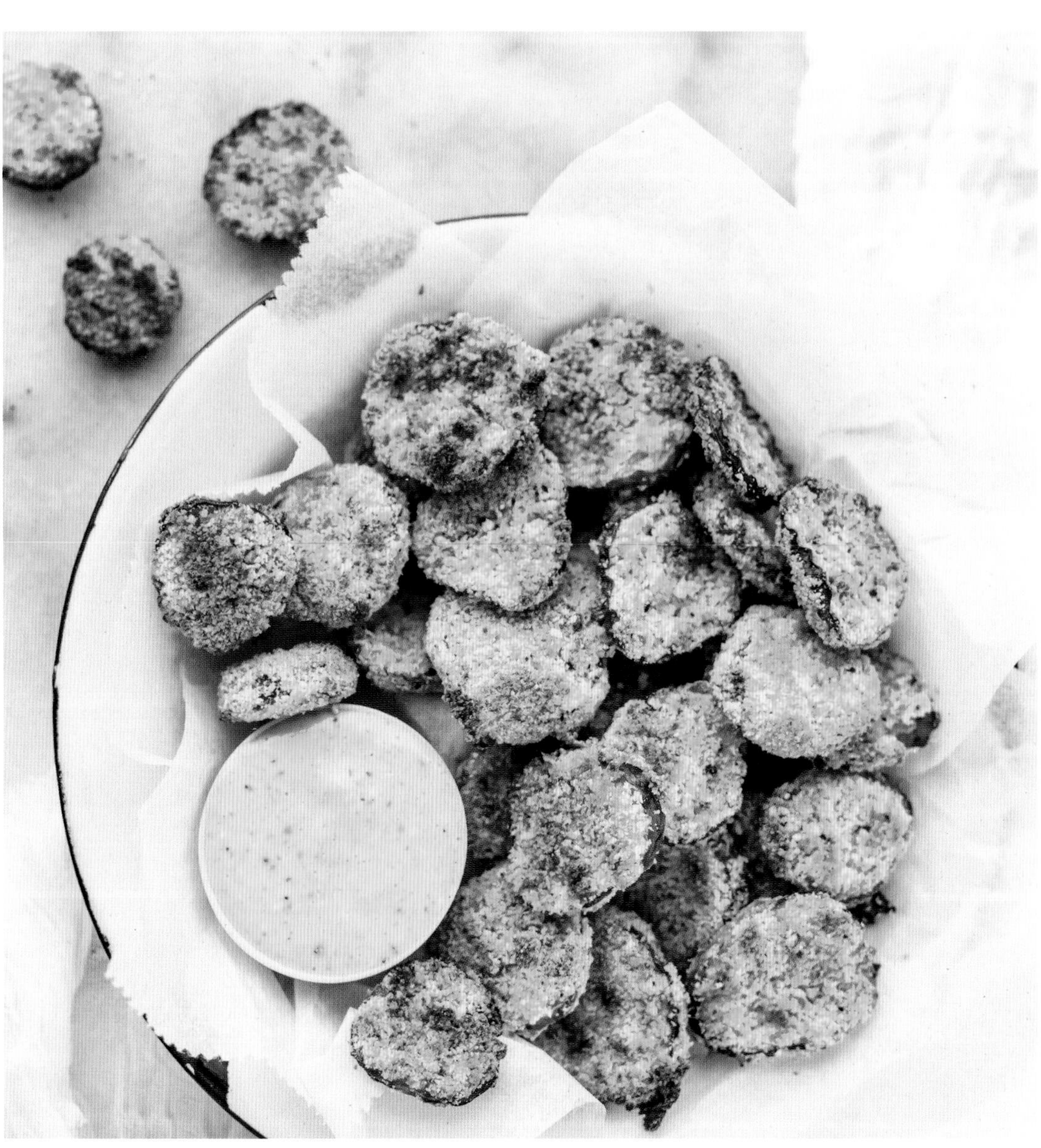

PICKLES

1 large egg

1 tablespoon (15 ml) canned unsweetened coconut milk

1 cup (96 g) almond flour

2 tablespoons (8 g) nutritional yeast

1½ teaspoons sea salt

1 teaspoon garlic powder

1 teaspoon black pepper

2 cups (400 g) no-sugar-added pickle slices

BOOM BOOM FRY SAUCE

1 cup (240 g) Mayo (page 28) or compliant mayonnaise

2 tablespoons (20 g) grated onion

2 tablespoons (30 g) no-sugar-added chopped pickles

2 tablespoons (30 g) no-sugar-added ketchup

1 tablespoon (15 ml) pickle juice

1½ teaspoons yellow mustard

½ teaspoon black pepper

¼ teaspoon garlic powder

¼ teaspoon paprika

¼ teaspoon sea salt

AIR FRYER VERSION

1. Preheat the air fryer to 390°F (198°C).
2. In a small bowl, beat together the egg and coconut milk.
3. In a separate small bowl, mix together the almond flour, nutritional yeast, salt, garlic powder, and pepper.
4. Place the pickles on a paper towel and pat dry. Dip each pickle slice in the egg mixture, then the almond flour mixture. Set aside on a plate or cutting board.
5. Working in two batches, place the pickle slices in the air fryer basket in a single layer and cook until golden brown, 8 to 10 minutes. Remove to a plate and repeat with the remaining pickles.
6. Serve with the Boom Boom Fry Sauce.

OVEN VERSION

1. Preheat the oven to 450°F (230°C or gas mark 8) and line a large baking sheet with parchment paper.
2. Follow steps 2 through 4 in the Air Fryer Version.
3. Place the pickles on the prepared baking sheet and bake until golden and crispy, about 15 minutes.

BOOM BOOM FRY SAUCE

1. Place the mayo in a wide-mouth mason jar or medium bowl.
2. Add the onion, pickles, ketchup, pickle juice, mustard, pepper, garlic powder, paprika, and salt.
3. Mix together with a spoon. Cap the jar and refrigerate for up to 1 week.

Creamy Green Chili-Chicken Dip

Dress up your veggie sticks with this creamy, slightly spicy dip. It's great for tailgating, backyard BBQs, and holiday gatherings.

SQUEAKY CLEAN PALEO / KETO PALEO / TRADITIONAL PALEO

Makes: 6 to 8 servings / **Prep Time:** 5 minutes / **Total Time:** 40 minutes

- 3 large (6 ounces [168 g]) boneless, skinless chicken breasts
- ½ cup (80 g) chopped onion
- ⅓ cup (50 g) diced tomatoes
- ⅓ cup (80 g) Mayo (page 28) or compliant mayonnaise
- 1 can (4 ounces [112 g]) green chiles, drained
- ¼ cup (16 g) nutritional yeast
- 2 tablespoons (30 ml) canned unsweetened coconut milk
- 1 tablespoon (6 g) arrowroot powder or almond flour if Keto
- 1 teaspoon ground cumin
- ½ teaspoon granulated garlic
- Sea salt, to taste
- ¼ teaspoon onion powder
- ¼ teaspoon black pepper

1. Preheat the oven to 350°F (180°C or gas mark 4). Spray a 10-inch (25 cm) cast-iron skillet or an 8 by 8-inch (20 by 20 cm) baking dish with olive oil cooking spray.
2. Place the chicken in a large pot of water to cover and bring to a boil over medium-high heat. Once the water is boiling, reduce the heat to low and cover with a lid. Cook until the chicken has reached an internal temperature of 160°F (71°C), about 15 minutes.
3. Remove the chicken to a cutting board and shred using one or two forks.
4. Transfer the chicken to a large bowl along with the chopped onion, tomatoes, mayo, green chiles, nutritional yeast, coconut milk, arrowroot, cumin, garlic, salt, onion powder, and pepper. Mix together with a spoon until well combined.
5. Add the chicken mixture to the prepared skillet or baking dish and smooth the top.
6. Bake until bubbling, 20 to 25 minutes.

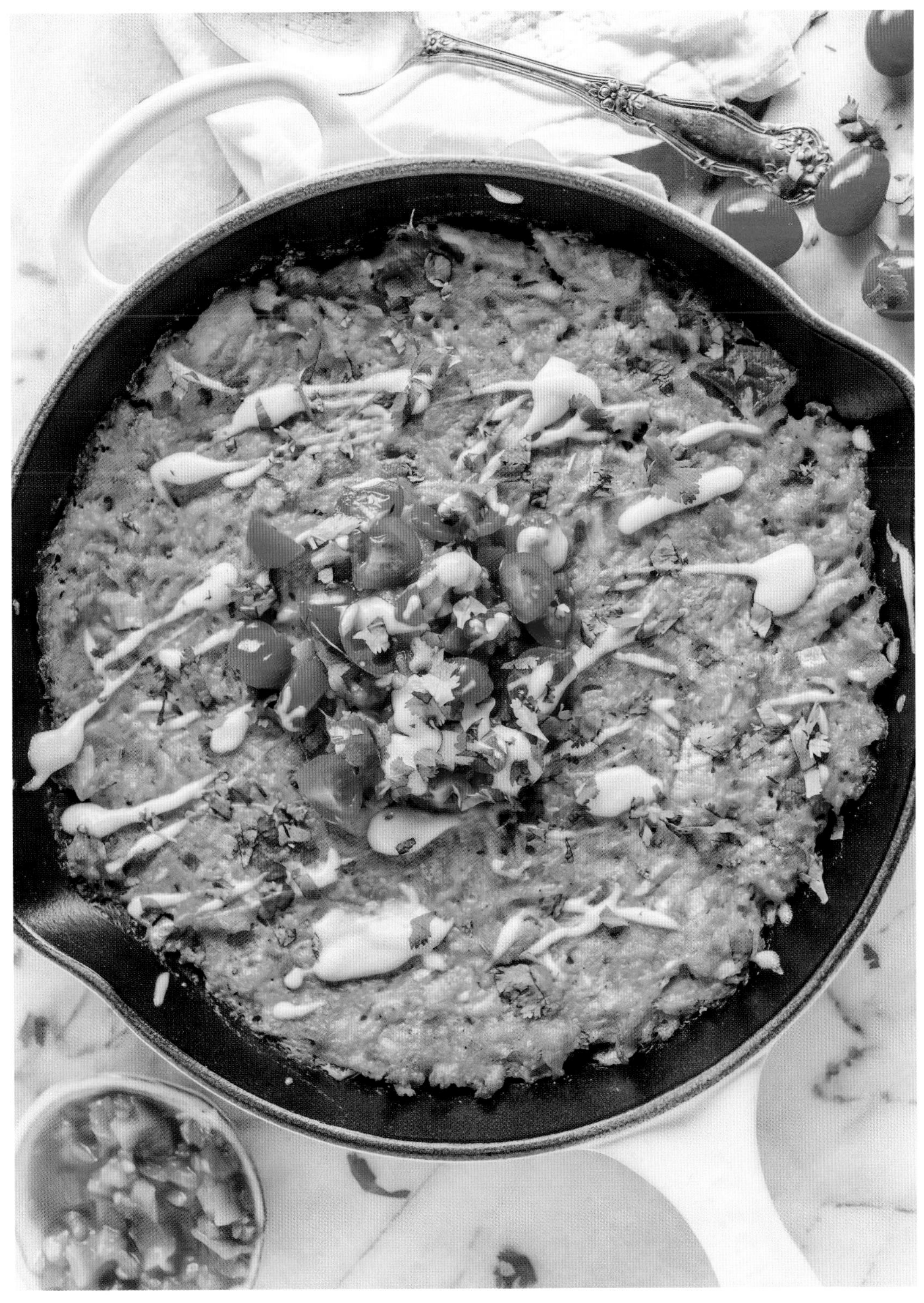

Twice-Baked Taco Sweet Potatoes

These twice-baked sweet potatoes are filled with all the flavors of Taco Tuesday. They can be served not only as an appetizer but also as a main dish.

SQUEAKY CLEAN PALEO / TRADITIONAL PALEO

Makes: 8 servings / **Prep Time:** 10 minutes / **Total Time:** 1 hour 20 minutes

---

4 large sweet potatoes, scrubbed
1 tablespoon (15 ml) olive oil
¼ cup (40 g) chopped onion
1 pound (454 g) 90/10 ground beef
2 tablespoons (30 ml) canned unsweetened coconut milk
2 tablespoons (8 g) nutritional yeast
1¼ teaspoons chili powder
1 teaspoon ground cumin
½ teaspoon onion powder
½ teaspoon garlic powder
¼ teaspoon dried oregano
¼ teaspoon sea salt
1 avocado, peeled, pitted, and diced, for garnish
Compliant salsa, for garnish

---

1. Preheat the oven to 375°F (190°C or gas mark 5). Pierce the potatoes several times with a fork. Set on a baking sheet and bake until tender, about 60 minutes.
2. Meanwhile, heat the olive oil in a large skillet over medium-high heat. Add the onion and cook until translucent, 4 to 5 minutes. Add the ground beef and cook until browned, 5 to 7 minutes.
3. Split the potatoes lengthwise and remove the insides of the sweet potatoes, transferring to a medium bowl. Reserve the skins for later.
4. To the flesh of the sweet potatoes, add the cooked ground beef and onions, along with the coconut milk, nutritional yeast, chili powder, cumin, onion powder, garlic powder, oregano, and salt. Mix together until completely combined.
5. Spoon the filling back into the potato skins and place on the baking sheet.
6. Return the potatoes to the oven and bake until golden brown, about 15 minutes.
7. Top each potato skin with avocado and salsa.

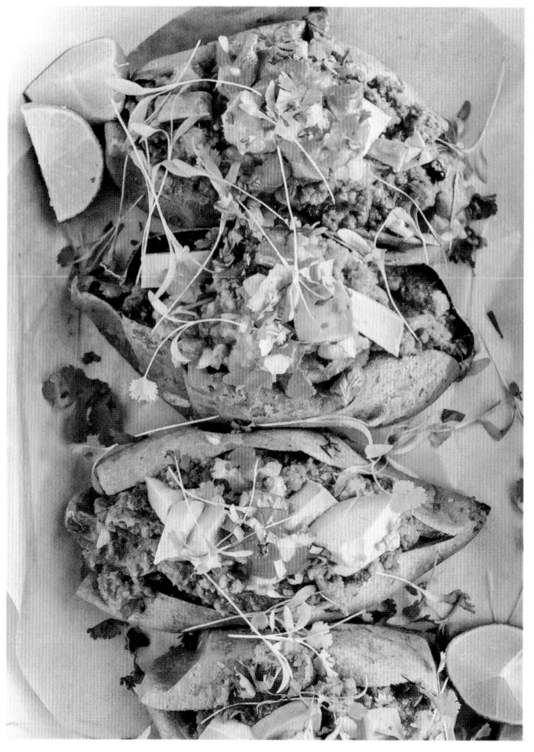

Mango and Pineapple Salsa

You get a little bit of sweet and a little bit of savory with this salsa that's perfect for dipping homemade tostones (see page 47) or sweet potato chips. It's also the perfect addition to salads and cooked chicken or fish. Tajin is a Mexican seasoning that is perfect on fruit and protein. You can find it in most grocery stores in the specialty Hispanic or Latin foods aisle.

SQUEAKY CLEAN PALEO / TRADITIONAL PALEO

Makes: 5 cups (1200 g) / **Prep Time:** 5 minutes / **Total Time:** 10 minutes

3½ cups (543 g) diced pineapple
1½ cups (263 g) diced mango
1 small red onion, diced
Juice of 1 lime
3 tablespoons (3 g) coarsely chopped cilantro
¾ teaspoon Tajin seasoning
Sea salt, to taste
¼ teaspoon black pepper

1. In a large bowl, gently combine the pineapple, mango, and onion.
2. Add the lime juice, cilantro, Tajin seasoning, salt, and pepper. Combine everything with a spoon until well mixed.
3. Serve immediately. The salsa will keep for up to 4 days if refrigerated in an airtight container.

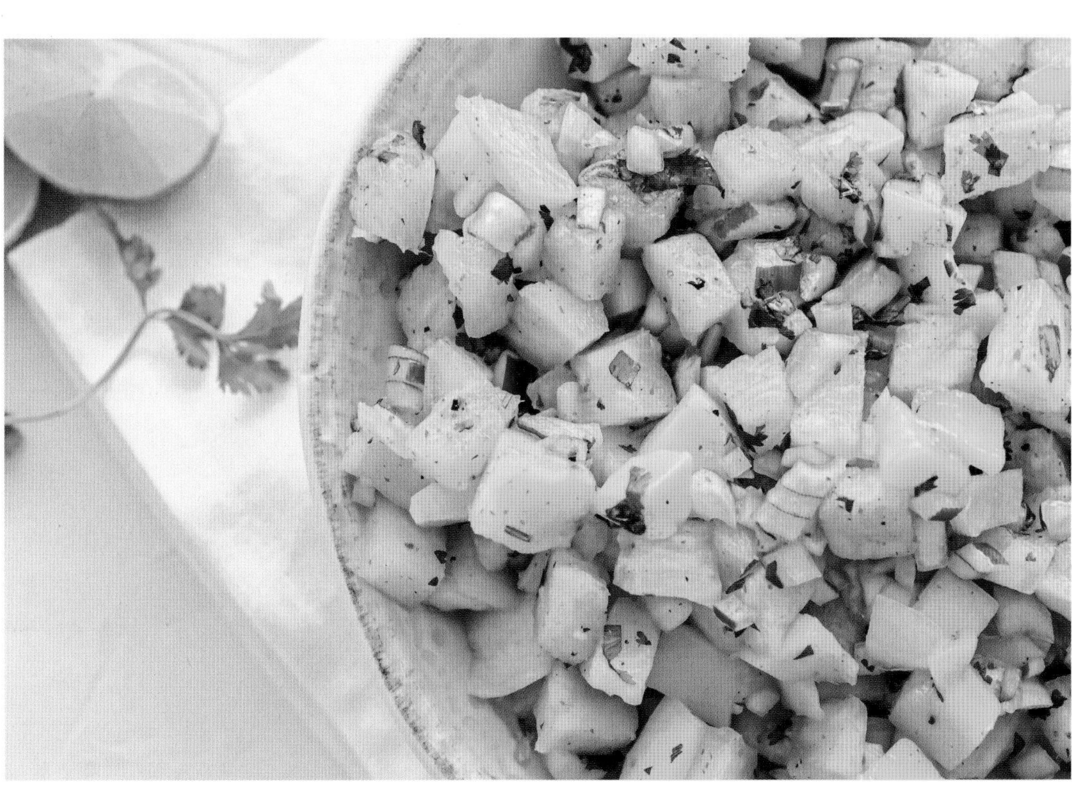

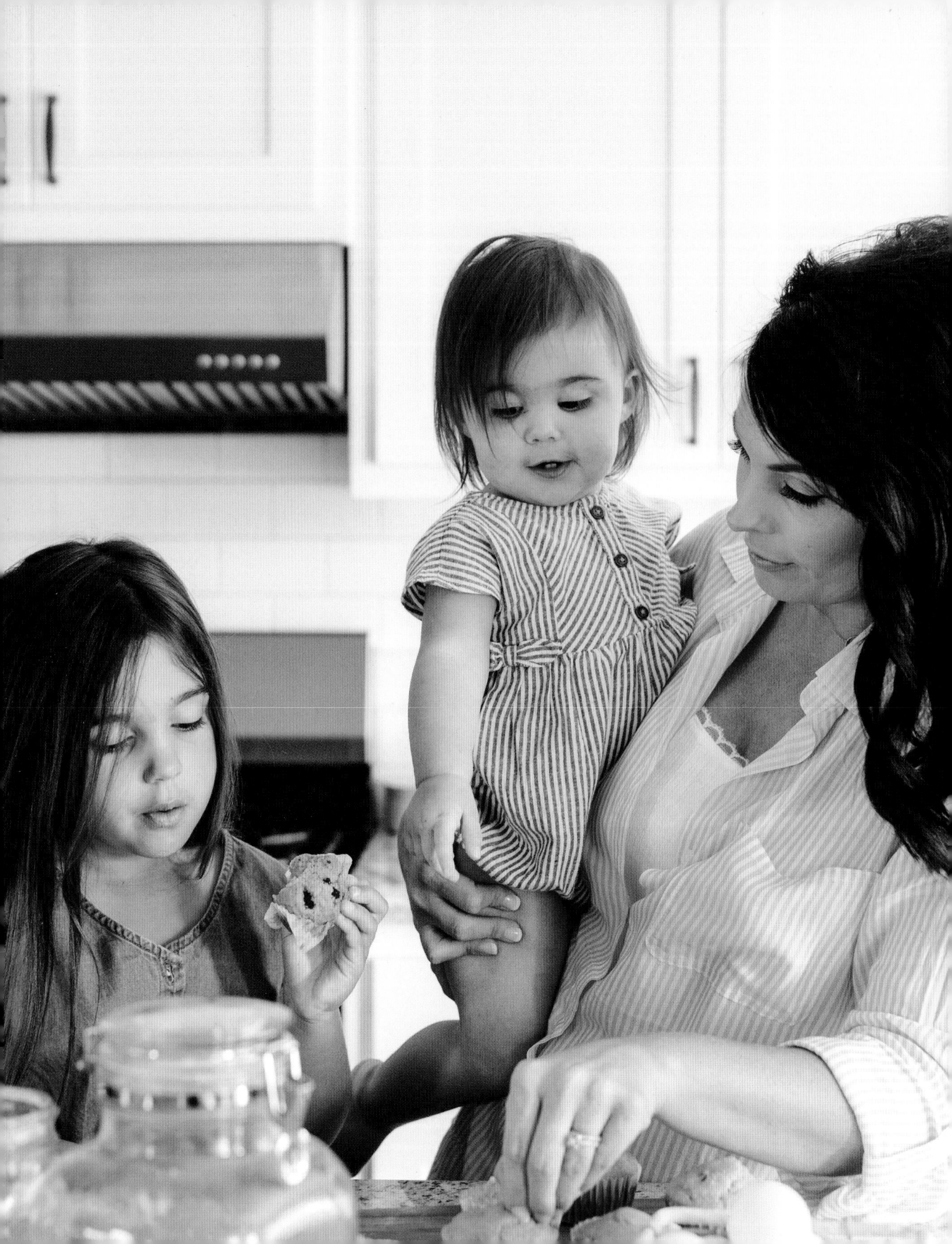

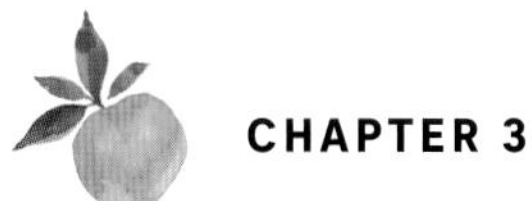

CHAPTER 3

Breakfast

I'm one of those Southern mommas who not only cooks a big delicious breakfast on Saturday and Sunday mornings, but I've also been known to serve it two or three times during the week for dinner. My family absolutely loves when I make breakfast, and they don't care what meal it's for. I find that breakfast dishes are quick to whip up, and they can also save money in your budget. Eggs serve as a great, cheap protein option that can be used in many ways—but they don't have to be boring.

Red Pepper and Sausage Frittata

When all else fails, make a frittata. They are seriously so simple and versatile and can be used as breakfast, lunch, or dinner. The flavors in this red pepper and sausage frittata are simple yet bursting with taste. It's a great meal-prep option and can serve as an easy breakfast or lunch during the week.

SQUEAKY CLEAN PALEO / KETO PALEO / TRADITIONAL PALEO

Makes: 8 servings / **Prep Time:** 10 minutes / **Total Time:** 40 minutes

1 tablespoon (14 g) ghee
½ sweet yellow onion, chopped
1 small red bell pepper, seeded and finely chopped
2 small cloves garlic, minced
1 pound (454 g) compliant ground sausage
2 tablespoons (8 g) nutritional yeast
¾ teaspoon sea salt
¼ teaspoon black pepper
¼ teaspoon paprika
8 large eggs
2 tablespoons (30 ml) canned unsweetened coconut milk
1 small avocado, peeled, pitted, and sliced
Compliant salsa, for serving

1. Preheat the oven to 350°F (180°C or gas mark 4). Spray a cast-iron skillet with olive oil cooking spray.
2. Heat the ghee in the skillet over medium heat until the ghee sizzles.
3. Add the onion, bell pepper, and garlic to the skillet. Cook until tender, about 4 minutes.
4. Add the sausage, nutritional yeast, salt, black pepper, and paprika. Combine the mixture with a spoon, breaking up the sausage. Cook until the sausage is cooked through and no longer pink, 6 to 7 minutes.
5. Meanwhile, in a large bowl, whisk together the eggs and coconut milk.
6. Pour the egg mixture on top of everything in the skillet. Make sure the mixture is spread evenly for even cooking.
7. Transfer the skillet to the oven and bake until the middle of the frittata is set, 25 to 30 minutes. (To test, stick a toothpick in the middle of the frittata and if it comes out clean, it is ready.)
8. Garnish with the avocado slices and a spoonful of salsa.

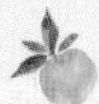

RECIPE NOTES

If you don't have a cast-iron skillet, transfer the sausage mixture to an 8 by 8-inch (20 by 20 cm) clear baking dish coated with olive oil cooking spray. Pour the egg mixture on top.

Breakfast Stuffed Peppers

Stuffed peppers aren't just for dinner, especially when the savory ground beef is mixed with fluffy scrambled eggs. I add my own special touch with a drizzle of homemade avocado-ranch.

SQUEAKY CLEAN PALEO / KETO PALEO / TRADITIONAL PALEO

Makes: 6 peppers / **Prep Time:** 10 minutes / **Total Time:** 30 minutes

3 multicolor bell peppers, halved and seeded
1 tablespoon (15 ml) olive oil
1 clove garlic, minced
1 pound (454 g) 90/10 ground beef
6 large eggs
2 tablespoons (30 ml) canned unsweetened coconut milk
2 tablespoons (8 g) nutritional yeast
1 tablespoon (15 ml) lime juice
½ teaspoon sea salt
¼ teaspoon black pepper
1 cup Ranch Dressing (page 30)
1 small avocado, peeled and pitted
Fresh coarsely chopped parsley or cilantro, for garnish

1. Preheat the oven to 400°F (200°C or gas mark 6) and grease a baking sheet with olive oil.
2. Place the peppers cut-side up on the baking sheet. Bake until tender, about 20 minutes.
3. Meanwhile, heat the olive oil and garlic in a large skillet over medium-high heat.
4. Add the ground beef and use a wooden spoon to break it up. Cook until brown and no longer pink, 6 to 7 minutes.
5. Pour the beef into a bowl and set aside.
6. In a medium bowl, whisk together the eggs, coconut milk, nutritional yeast, lime juice, salt, and pepper.
7. Pour the egg mixture into the skillet and reduce the heat to low. Using a wooden spoon or spatula, move the eggs back and forth and cook until fluffy, about 5 minutes.
8. Add back the cooked ground beef and fold together with the spoon until combined.
9. Remove the peppers from the oven and fill each with the egg-beef mixture.
10. Return the peppers to the oven and bake for 10 minutes more.
11. Meanwhile, in a wide-mouth mason jar or small bowl, add the ranch and avocado. Using an immersion blender, blend together until creamy. (You may also do this in a regular blender.)
12. Allow the peppers to cool slightly before plating, drizzled with the avocado-ranch and topped with parsley.
13. If there is dressing left, add to a mason jar and cap with a lid. Will keep in the refrigerator for a day or two. Due to the nature of the avocado, it may turn brown if stored any longer.

BLT Eggs Benny over Crispy Tostones

These BLT eggs Benedict are perfect for a weekend breakfast. They're layered with the traditional BLT toppings and hollandaise sauce, but crispy fried plantains take the place of the typical English muffin.

SQUEAKY CLEAN PALEO / TRADITIONAL PALEO

Makes: 4 servings / **Prep Time:** 10 minutes / **Total Time:** 30 minutes

BACON AND TOSTONES

4 slices compliant bacon
2 green plantains, peeled and cut into 1-inch (2.5 cm) chunks (omit if Keto)
1 cup (240 g) coconut oil, divided
Sea salt

HOLLANDAISE SAUCE

3 large egg yolks
1 tablespoon (15 ml) lemon juice
½ teaspoon compliant hot sauce
½ teaspoon sea salt
¼ teaspoon cayenne pepper
½ cup (120 g) ghee, melted

EGGS AND ASSEMBLY

2 teaspoons white vinegar
1 teaspoon kosher salt
4 large eggs, cold
2 cups (60 g) arugula salad mix
4 large slices tomato
Microgreens

BACON AND TOSTONES

1. Preheat the oven to 400°F (200°C or gas mark 6).
2. Place the bacon on a baking sheet.
3. Bake for 15 to 20 minutes, or until desired doneness.
4. Transfer to a paper towel to drain.
5. Meanwhile, heat ½ cup (120 g) of the coconut oil in a large skillet over medium-high heat. Place the plantains in the oil and fry until browned on both sides, about 4 minutes on each side.
6. Remove the plantains from the skillet, placing them one at a time in between two pieces of parchment paper. Use a flat surface, such as the bottom of a glass, to press down and flatten the plantains. Set aside until they're all flattened.
7. Heat the remaining ½ cup (120 g) oil in the skillet. When hot, return the flattened plantains and fry until crispy, 1 minute on each side.
8. Remove the crispy tostones to a plate and sprinkle with salt.

HOLLANDAISE SAUCE

1. Add the egg yolks, lemon juice, hot sauce, salt, and cayenne pepper to a mason jar.
2. Add a little bit of the ghee to the mason jar and use an immersion blender on high speed to start blending together. Slowly pour the rest of the ghee into the jar as you are blending. The sauce will thicken and become a creamy pale yellow.

RECIPE NOTES

If you do not have an immersion blender, do all the steps with a blender, pouring the ghee through the hole in the cap.

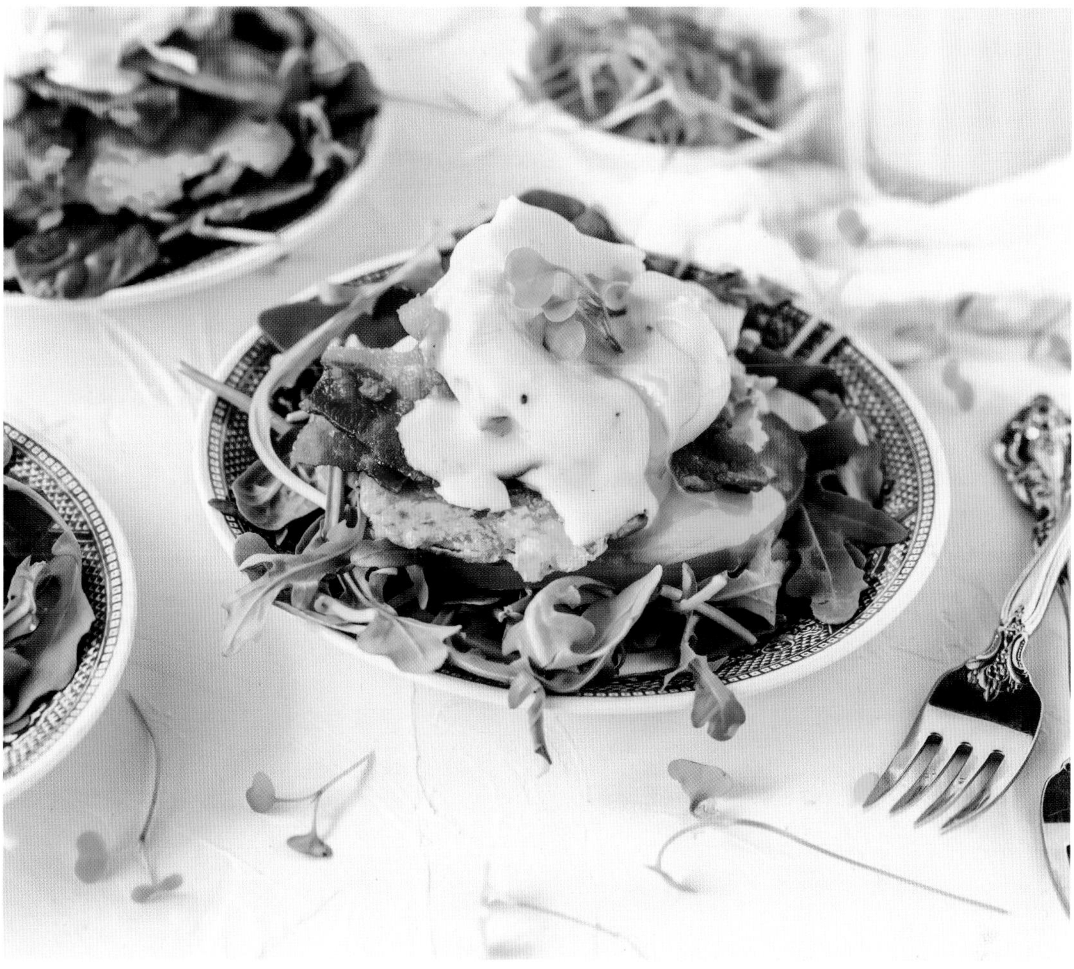

EGGS AND ASSEMBLY

1. Bring a large skillet of water to a gentle boil with the vinegar and salt.
2. Meanwhile, crack the cold eggs into custard cups or small bowls (1 egg per cup).
3. Carefully slide or slowly pour each egg into the water, one at a time.
4. Cover with a lid and remove from the heat. Set aside for 3 minutes.
5. Use a slotted spoon to remove each egg to a paper towel–lined plate to drain the excess water.
6. To assemble, add ½ cup (15 g) arugula to each of 4 plates.
7. Place a tomato slice over the arugula, followed by 2 tostones, a slice of bacon, and 1 poached egg. Pour the hollandaise sauce over everything. Garnish with microgreens and serve.

Loaded Breakfast Sweet Potato Fries

Who says you can't have loaded fries for breakfast? This recipe is simply genius and will make you excited to wake up just so you can have it. Get the fries in the oven first thing, and the rest of the recipe will be smooth sailing, I promise.

SQUEAKY CLEAN PALEO / TRADITIONAL PALEO

Makes: 4 servings / **Prep Time:** 15 minutes / **Total Time:** 45 minutes

SWEET POTATO FRIES

4 medium sweet potatoes, cut into ¼-inch (6 mm)-thick fries
1½ tablespoons (23 ml) olive oil
½ teaspoon sea salt
¼ teaspoon black pepper

SAUSAGE

1 tablespoon (15 ml) olive oil
2 cloves garlic, minced
1½ pounds (680 g) ground breakfast sausage (no sugar added)
¼ teaspoon sea salt
¼ teaspoon black pepper

EGGS AND ASSEMBLY

2 teaspoons white vinegar
1 teaspoon kosher salt
4 large eggs, cold
Mac's Awesome Sauce (page 31)
Fresh coarsely chopped parsley, for garnish

SWEET POTATO FRIES

1. Preheat the oven to 425°F (220°C or gas mark 7) and line a baking sheet with parchment paper.
2. Put the cut fries in a large bowl and toss with the olive oil, salt, and pepper until evenly coated.
3. Transfer to the prepared baking sheet, making sure they are not overcrowded.
4. Bake until brown and crisp on the bottom, about 20 minutes. Flip and cook for an additional 10 minutes, or until desired crispiness.

SAUSAGE

1. Heat the olive oil and garlic in a large skillet over medium heat.
2. Add the sausage, salt, and pepper and cook, breaking up the sausage using a wooden spoon, until browned and no longer pink inside, 6 to 7 minutes.

EGGS AND ASSEMBLY

1. If you are not a fan of poached eggs, simply substitute a fried egg, cooked to your liking. For poached eggs, bring a large skillet of water to a gentle boil with the vinegar and salt.
2. Meanwhile, crack the cold eggs into custard cups or small bowls (1 egg per cup).
3. Carefully slide or slowly pour each egg into the water, one at a time.
4. Cover with a lid. Set aside for 3 minutes.
5. Use a slotted spoon to remove each egg to a paper towel-lined plate to drain the excess water.
6. To assemble, divide the sweet potato fries among 4 bowls.
7. Put ¼ cup (60 g) of the sausage mixture on top of the fries, along with a poached egg. Drizzle with Mac's Awesome Sauce and sprinkle with parsley.

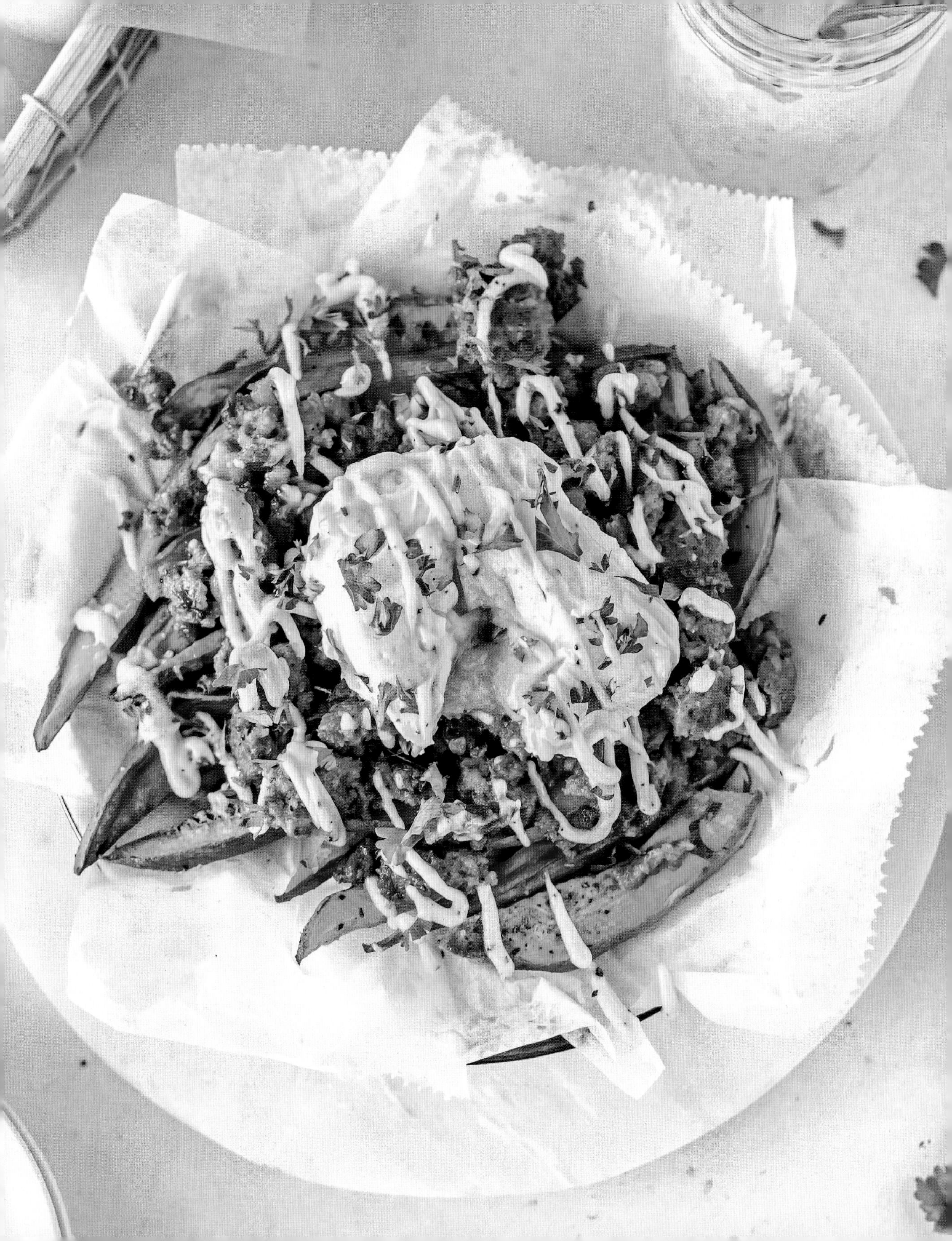

Chicken Fajita Egg Cups

These traditional egg muffin cups are loaded with chicken and infused with fajita seasoning. They're great for grab-and-go breakfasts or quick snacks. Cook an extra chicken breast the next time you're at the stove, and these will be a cinch to make in the morning. Bonus: They freeze very well!

SQUEAKY CLEAN PALEO / KETO PALEO / TRADITIONAL PALEO

Makes: 12 egg cups / **Prep Time:** 5 minutes / **Total Time:** 30 minutes

12 large eggs
1 tablespoon (15 ml) canned unsweetened coconut milk
1 large cooked chicken breast (skin removed), cubed
½ cup (80 g) diced yellow onion
1 small green bell pepper, seeded and finely diced
¼ cup (60 ml) compliant salsa
1 tablespoon (4 g) nutritional yeast (optional)
½ teaspoon chili powder
½ teaspoon sea salt
¼ teaspoon black pepper
¼ teaspoon ground cumin
¼ teaspoon garlic powder
¼ teaspoon paprika

1. Preheat the oven to 375°F (190°C or gas mark 5) and coat a 12-cup muffin tin with olive oil cooking spray.
2. In a large bowl, whisk together the eggs and coconut milk until combined and smooth.
3. Add the chicken, onion, bell pepper, salsa, nutritional yeast (if using), chili powder, salt, black pepper, cumin, garlic powder, and paprika. Whisk until evenly combined.
4. Divide the mixture among the muffin cups.
5. Bake until the egg mixture is firm and no longer jiggles, 20 to 25 minutes.
6. Remove the egg muffins and let cool briefly before serving or completely before storing in the fridge.

Pot Roast Hash with Fried Eggs

This hearty breakfast dish is perfect for when you have leftover pot roast from a day or two earlier.

SQUEAKY CLEAN PALEO / TRADITIONAL PALEO

Makes: 5 servings / **Prep Time:** 5 minutes / **Total Time:** 30 minutes

- 2 tablespoons (28 g) ghee, divided
- 1½ cups (180 g) diced sweet potatoes, skin on
- ⅓ cup (53 g) finely chopped sweet onion
- 2 cloves garlic, minced
- 3 cups (420 g) shredded Pot Roast (page 144)
- 1 cup (70 g) shredded Brussels sprouts
- 5 large eggs
- ½ teaspoon sea salt
- ¼ teaspoon black pepper

1. Preheat the oven to 450°F (230°C or gas mark 8).
2. Heat 1 tablespoon (14 g) of the ghee in a cast-iron skillet over medium-high heat until the ghee sizzles.
3. Add the sweet potatoes, onion, and garlic. Cook, stirring, until the potatoes are tender, about 15 minutes.
4. Add the roast and Brussels sprouts. Stir everything together and simmer for 4 to 5 minutes.
5. Meanwhile, in another skillet, heat the remaining 1 tablespoon (14 g) ghee over medium-high heat until the ghee sizzles.
6. Break the eggs into the skillet, leaving room between each. Sprinkle with the salt and pepper. Reduce the heat to low. Cook until desired doneness, 2 to 3 minutes.
7. Add the eggs over the top of the pot roast hash and serve immediately.

RECIPE NOTES

If you don't have leftover pot roast, you can also cook your roast overnight in the slow cooker so it's ready for breakfast.

Pineapple-Mango Chia Seed Pudding

This chia seed pudding is a great alternative to oatmeal. It can be made the night before so it's ready to grab the next morning. All you'll have left to do is puree the pineapple and mango topping.

TRADITIONAL PALEO

Makes: 2 servings / **Prep Time:** 5 minutes / **Total Time:** 45 minutes

CHIA SEED PUDDING

- 4 tablespoons (36 g) chia seeds, divided
- 2 cups (480 ml) unsweetened almond milk, divided
- 2 teaspoons honey or other sweetener of choice, divided (optional)
- ½ teaspoon pure vanilla extract, divided

PINEAPPLE AND MANGO TOPPING

- ½ cup (83 g) frozen pineapple chunks
- ½ cup (88 g) frozen mango chunks
- 2 tablespoons (30 ml) canned unsweetened coconut milk
- Toasted unsweetened coconut flakes, for garnish

CHIA SEED PUDDING

1. In two separate wide-mouth mason jars, add 2 tablespoons (18 g) of the chia seeds to each jar.
2. To each jar, pour 1 cup (240 ml) of the almond milk along with 1 teaspoon of the honey and ¼ teaspoon of the vanilla.
3. Mix together with a spoon until combined.
4. Screw the lids on and let sit for 4 to 5 minutes. Give them one more big shake to make sure everything is combined.
5. Refrigerate for 30 minutes or overnight for best results.

PINEAPPLE AND MANGO TOPPING

1. To a blender or food processor, add the pineapple, mango, and coconut milk. Blend on high speed until combined.
2. If the mixture is too thick, add more coconut milk to thin it out.
3. Divide between the two chia seed puddings and garnish with the coconut flakes.

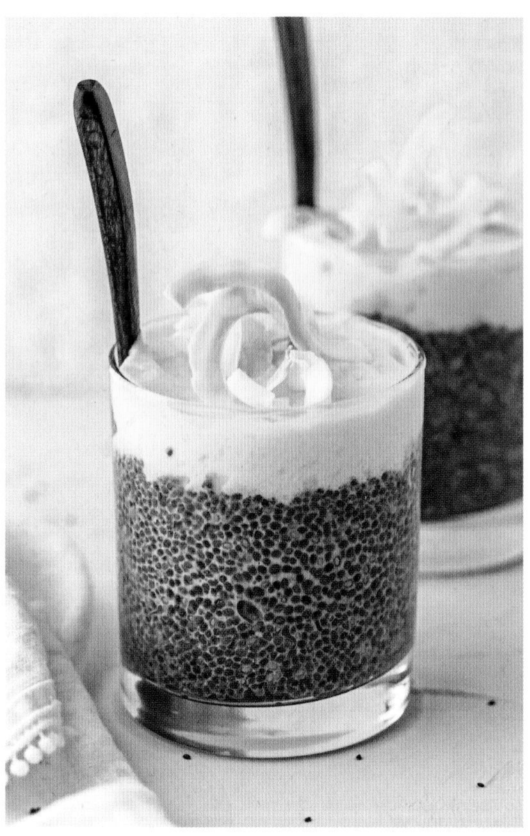

Paleo Granola

Store-bought granolas can be very non-Paleo friendly. They're also expensive! My version uses a variety of nuts infused with cinnamon and honey, baked until crispy golden brown, and it's so simple to make. Eat it as a snack or add almond milk to make the perfect Paleo cereal.

TRADITIONAL PALEO

Makes: 8 servings / **Prep Time:** 10 minutes / **Total Time:** 40 minutes

- ½ cup (60 g) chopped pecans
- ½ cup (60 g) chopped walnuts
- ½ cup (55 g) sliced almonds
- ½ cup (40 g) unsweetened coconut flakes
- ⅓ cup (45 g) raw cashew halves
- ¼ cup (37 g) unsweetened raisins, dried blueberries, or cranberries
- 1 teaspoon ground cinnamon
- ½ teaspoon sea salt
- ½ cup (170 g) raw honey
- ¼ cup (60 g) coconut oil
- 1 teaspoon pure vanilla extract

1. Preheat the oven to 300°F (150°C or gas mark 2) and line a large baking sheet with parchment paper.
2. In a large bowl, combine the pecans, walnuts, almonds, coconut flakes, cashews, dried fruit, cinnamon, and salt.
3. In a glass measuring cup, add the honey, coconut oil, and vanilla. Heat in the microwave for 30 seconds. Stir to combine.
4. Pour the warm liquid over the nut mixture and stir together until everything is well combined and coated.
5. Spread the mixture evenly on the prepared baking sheet. Bake until it is golden and crispy, about 20 minutes.
6. Remove from the oven and let cool on the baking sheet for 10 minutes.
7. Break the granola with your hands or a fork.
8. Cool completely and store in an airtight container in a dry place for up to 6 months.

RECIPE NOTES

You can freeze granola, wrapped tightly in plastic wrap and/or in a resealable freezer bag.

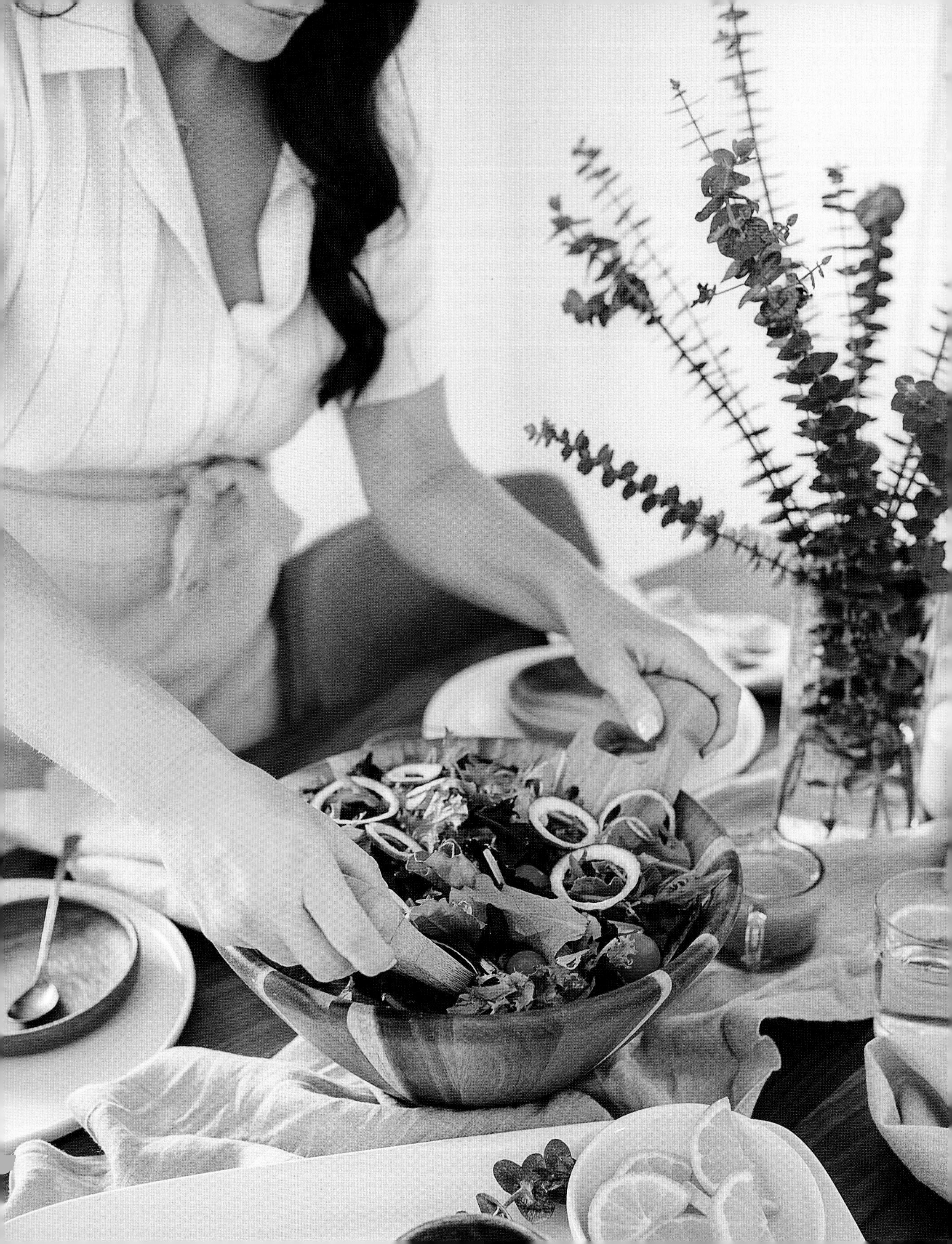

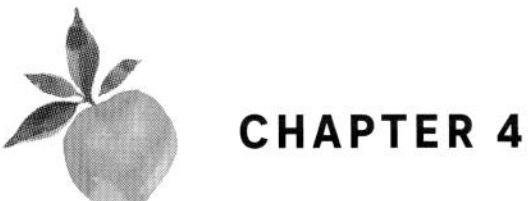

CHAPTER 4

Salads

Sometimes a big beautiful salad is what will set my heart on fire. In the warmer months, especially summer, I crave salad nonstop, whether it's my Spicy Shrimp Salad (page 76) or my Tuna Salad–Stuffed Avocados (page 84). Because boring lettuce and grilled chicken can get old real quick, I've developed healthy yet flavorful salads that are sure to chase all your blues away—no matter what season it is.

Taco Salad with Avocado Ranch

This quick and easy taco salad is filled with savory ground beef, lots of fresh veggies, and a heaping drizzle of homemade avocado ranch.

SQUEAKY CLEAN PALEO / KETO PALEO / TRADITIONAL PALEO

Makes: 4 to 6 servings / **Prep Time:** 6 minutes / **Total Time:** 25 minutes

---

TACO MEAT

1 tablespoon (15 ml) olive oil
1½ pounds (680 g) 90/10 ground beef
1 can (8 ounces [224 g]) no-sugar-added tomato sauce
1 tablespoon (6 g) chili powder
1½ teaspoons ground cumin
1 teaspoon paprika
1 teaspoon dried oregano
1 teaspoon black pepper
½ teaspoon sea salt
½ teaspoon garlic powder
¼ teaspoon onion powder

AVOCADO RANCH

1 cup (240 ml) Ranch Dressing (page 30)
1 avocado, peeled and pitted

SALAD

8 cups (240 g) lettuce of choice
1 cup (160 g) chopped red onion
1 cup (150 g) grape tomatoes, sliced
2 avocados, peeled, pitted, and sliced
4 tablespoons (36 g) sliced jalapeño
4 teaspoons (1 g) chopped cilantro
1 lime, quartered

TACO MEAT

1. Heat the olive oil in a large skillet over medium heat.
2. Add the ground beef and cook, using a wooden spoon to break up the meat, until it is brown and cooked through, about 7 minutes.
3. Add the tomato sauce, chili powder, cumin, paprika, oregano, pepper, salt, garlic powder, and onion powder. Stir to combine, then simmer over low heat for about 3 minutes.
4. Remove from the heat and set aside to cool.

AVOCADO RANCH

1. Add the ranch to a wide-mouth mason jar or medium bowl.
2. Add the avocado and blend together using an immersion blender until smooth. (You may also use a regular blender.)
3. If there is extra dressing, transfer to a jar with an airtight lid and refrigerate overnight. Due to the nature of the avocado, it may brown if not used within a day or two.

SALAD

1. Place 2 cups (60 g) lettuce in each of 4 bowls or plates and divide the taco meat among each salad. Divide the onion, tomatoes, avocados, and jalapeño evenly among the 4 salads. (Use a little less of everything if you're serving 6.)
2. Drizzle the salads with the avocado ranch and sprinkle with the cilantro. Add a lime wedge to each salad.

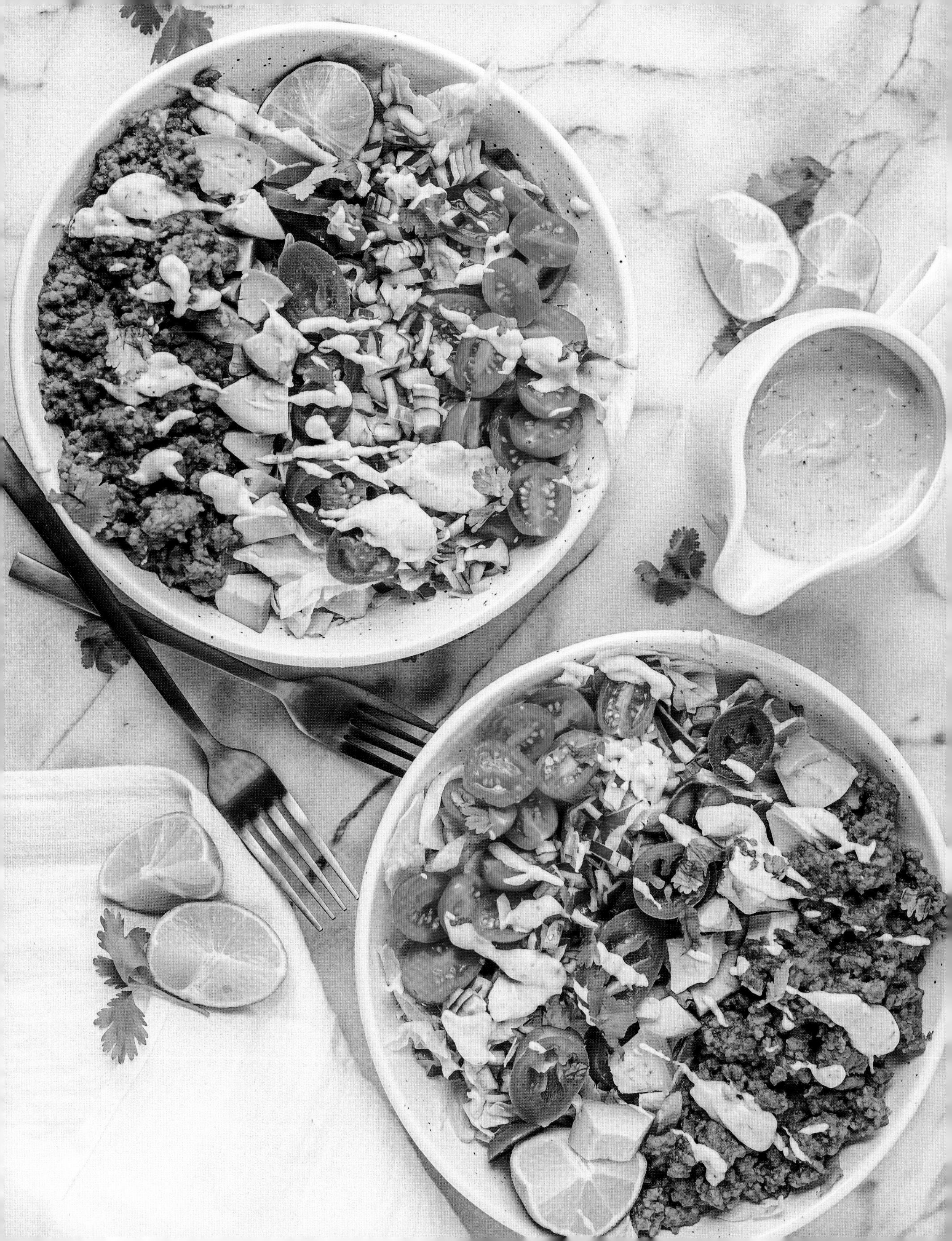

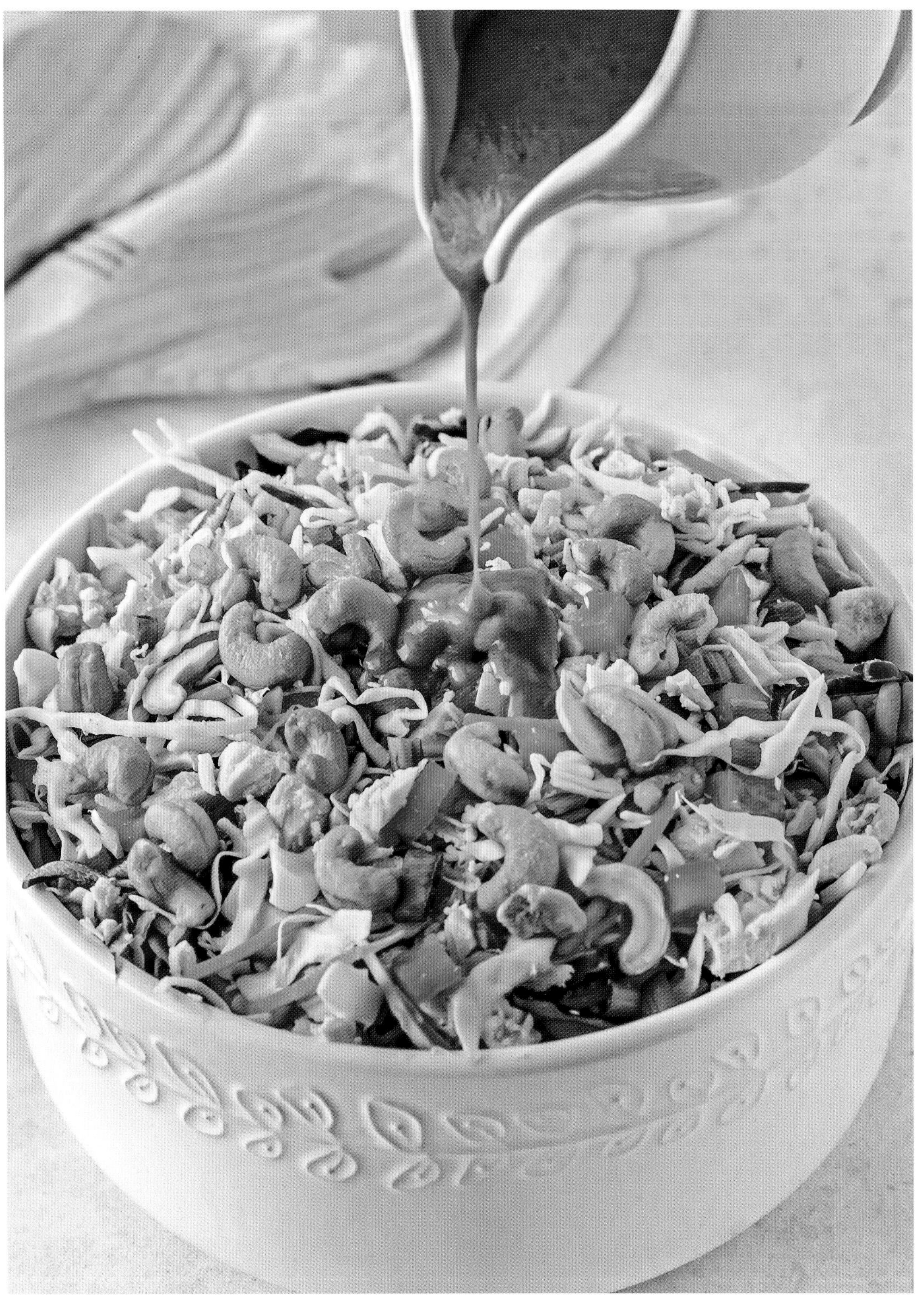

Thai Chicken Coleslaw with Almond Sauce

A spin on both the traditional creamy coleslaw and an Asian-style salad, this Thai Chicken Coleslaw gets doused in a luscious Paleo almond sauce and topped with cashews and scallions. This is the perfect salad for an outdoor BBQ or picnic.

SQUEAKY CLEAN PALEO / KETO PALEO / TRADITIONAL PALEO

Makes: 4 servings / **Prep Time:** 5 minutes / **Total Time:** 20 minutes

COLESLAW

3 medium (4 ounces [112 g]) boneless, skinless chicken breasts
1 bag (14 ounces [392 g]) plain coleslaw mix
½ cup (75 g) diced red bell pepper
⅓ cup (35 g) sliced scallions, plus more for garnish
¼ cup (30 g) halved cashews, plus more for garnish

ALMOND SAUCE

⅓ cup (85 g) all-natural, no-sugar-added almond butter
¼ cup (60 ml) extra-light olive oil
Juice of 1 lemon
3 tablespoons (45 ml) coconut aminos
1 tablespoon (15 ml) sesame oil
½ teaspoon rice vinegar
¼ teaspoon ground ginger
¼ teaspoon garlic powder
Sea salt and black pepper, if desired

COLESLAW

1. Place the chicken in a large pot of water to cover and bring to a boil over medium-high heat. Once the water is boiling, reduce the heat to low and cover with a lid. Simmer until the chicken reaches an internal temperature of 160°F (71°C), about 15 minutes.
2. Remove the chicken to a cutting board and shred using one or two forks. Allow to cool.
3. Meanwhile, put the coleslaw mix in a large bowl.
4. Add the bell pepper, scallions, cashews, and chicken. Toss to combine.

ALMOND SAUCE

1. Add the almond butter, olive oil, lemon juice, coconut aminos, sesame oil, vinegar, ginger, garlic powder, salt, and pepper to a blender. (You may also use an immersion blender.) Blend until smooth and creamy. If you are using an immersion blender, add all the ingredients to a wide-mouth mason jar, and blend until creamy and smooth, about 30 seconds.
2. Add the sauce to the coleslaw and mix together until well combined.
3. Serve garnished with the reserved scallions and cashews.

Spicy Shrimp Salad

This is no boring salad! Here, a mound of veggies gets topped with shrimp that's been cooked to perfection and tossed in spicy Bang Bang Sauce. It's quick enough for lunch and filling enough for dinner.

SQUEAKY CLEAN PALEO / KETO PALEO / TRADITIONAL PALEO

Makes: 4 servings / **Prep Time:** 10 minutes / **Total Time:** 25 minutes

1 tablespoon (15 ml) olive oil
1 pound (454 g) large peeled and deveined shrimp
½ cup (120 ml) Bang Bang Sauce (page 33)
6 to 8 cups (180 to 240 g) arugula and spinach mix (or lettuce of choice)
1 cup (150 g) halved grape tomatoes
¾ cup (120 g) sliced red onion
1 large avocado, peeled, pitted, and sliced
⅓ cup (40 g) slivered almonds
Crushed red pepper flakes, for garnish (optional)

1. Heat the olive oil in a large skillet over medium-high heat. Add the shrimp (they should sizzle when they hit the oil). Cook until the shrimp are pink or opaque and the tails curl, 4 to 5 minutes.
2. Transfer the shrimp to a paper towel–lined plate to absorb the excess oil.
3. Place the shrimp in a medium bowl and allow to cool. Toss with the Bang Bang Sauce until evenly coated.
4. Add the arugula and spinach mix to a serving dish. Assemble the salad by topping with the tomatoes, followed by the onion, spicy shrimp, avocado, and almonds. Sprinkle with a little bit of red pepper flakes, if desired.

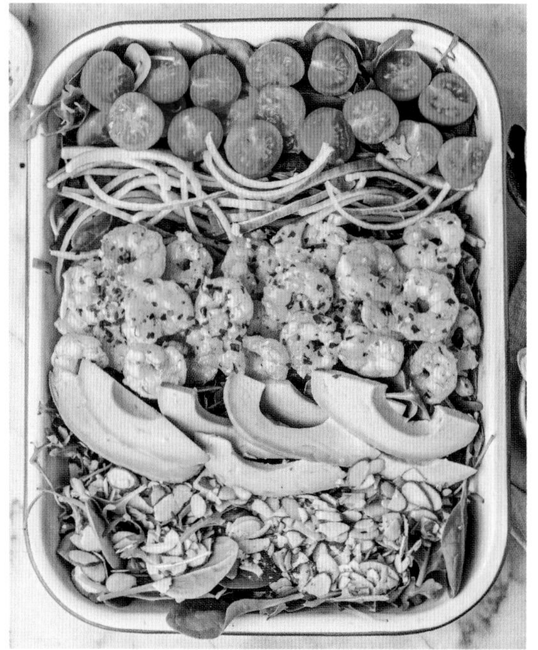

Chipotle Chicken Salad

This spin on the traditional chicken salad turns up the heat with cayenne pepper, chili powder, and green chiles. It has crunch from bell pepper and onion but is oh-so-creamy—and Paleo friendly! —with homemade mayo.

SQUEAKY CLEAN PALEO / KETO PALEO / TRADITIONAL PALEO

Makes: 4 servings / **Prep Time:** 10 minutes / **Total Time:** 15 to 20 minutes

4 medium boneless, skinless chicken breasts (4 ounces [112 g] each)
¾ cup (180 g) Mayo (page 28) or compliant mayonnaise
½ cup (75 g) plus 1 tablespoon (9 g) diced red bell pepper, divided
⅓ cup (53 g) diced onion
1 can (4 ounces [112 g]) green chiles, drained
1 teaspoon lime juice
1 teaspoon ground cumin
½ teaspoon chipotle chili powder
¼ teaspoon garlic powder
¼ teaspoon black pepper
¼ teaspoon sea salt
⅛ teaspoon cayenne pepper
Scallions

1. Place the chicken in a large pot of water to cover and bring to a boil over medium-high heat. Once the water is boiling, reduce the heat to low and cover with a lid. Simmer until the chicken reaches an internal temperature of 160°F (71°C), about 15 minutes.
2. Remove the chicken to a cutting board and allow to cool. Dice into small cubes.
3. Transfer the chicken to a large mixing bowl, along with the mayo, ½ cup (75 g) of the bell pepper, onion, green chiles, lime juice, cumin, chili powder, garlic powder, black pepper, salt, and cayenne.
4. Use a spoon to mix until well combined.
5. Garnish with the scallion and remaining 1 tablespoon (9 g) bell pepper.

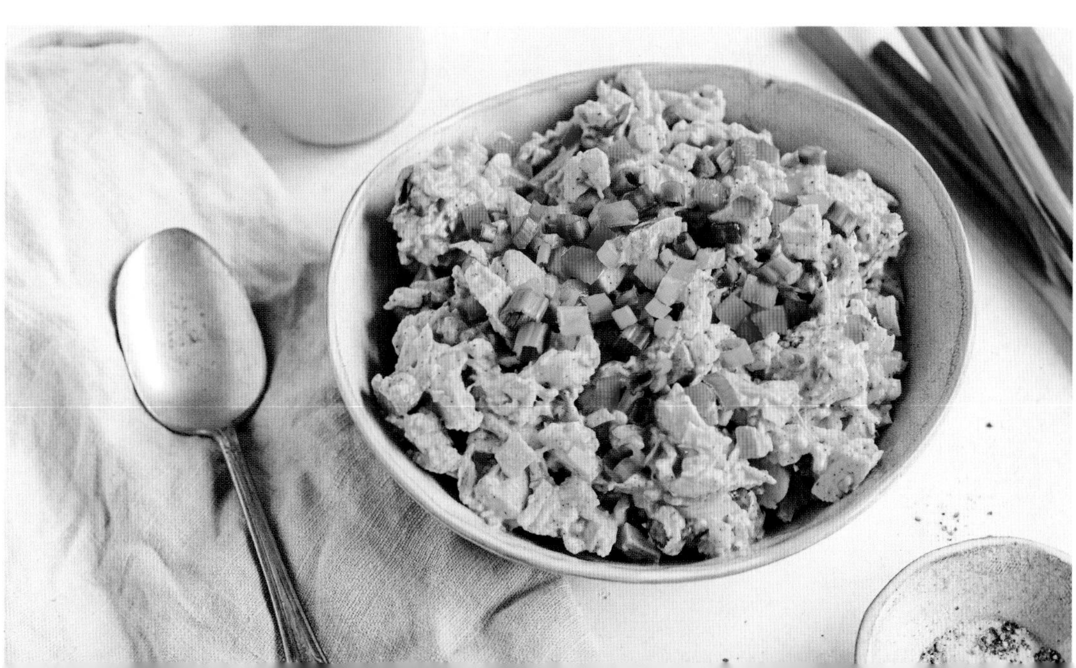

Cold Greek Zoodle Salad

Zoodles have never been more delicious than in this Greek-inspired salad that's filled with the flavors of the Mediterranean: artichoke hearts, olives, pepperoncini, red onions, and a tangy Greek vinaigrette. Serve it as a side dish to your main protein, such as chicken, or chop your protein and mix it right into the salad.

SQUEAKY CLEAN PALEO / KETO PALEO / TRADITIONAL PALEO

Makes: 4 servings / **Prep Time:** 15 minutes / **Total Time:** 20 minutes

---

- 3 large zucchini
- ½ jar (12 ounces [336 g]) artichoke hearts, drained and quartered
- ½ large red onion, sliced
- ¾ cup (115 g) halved cherry tomatoes
- ⅓ cup (35 g) pitted kalamata olives
- ⅓ cup (35 g) pepperoncini
- ½ cup (120 ml) Greek Dressing (page 37)
- Sea salt and black pepper, to taste

---

1. Cut the zucchini into noodle-shaped strands, also called "zoodles," using a spiralizing tool.
2. Place the spiralized zucchini into a large bowl and top with the artichoke hearts, onion, tomatoes, olives, and pepperoncini.
3. Whisk together the dressing. Pour over the zoodle mixture and toss to coat.
4. Serve immediately, or refrigerate in an air-tight container for up to 1 week.

RECIPE NOTES

You can find zucchini noodles in many grocery stores, but they're a bit pricey. If you go that route to save time, buy 4 to 4½ cups (480 to 540 g).

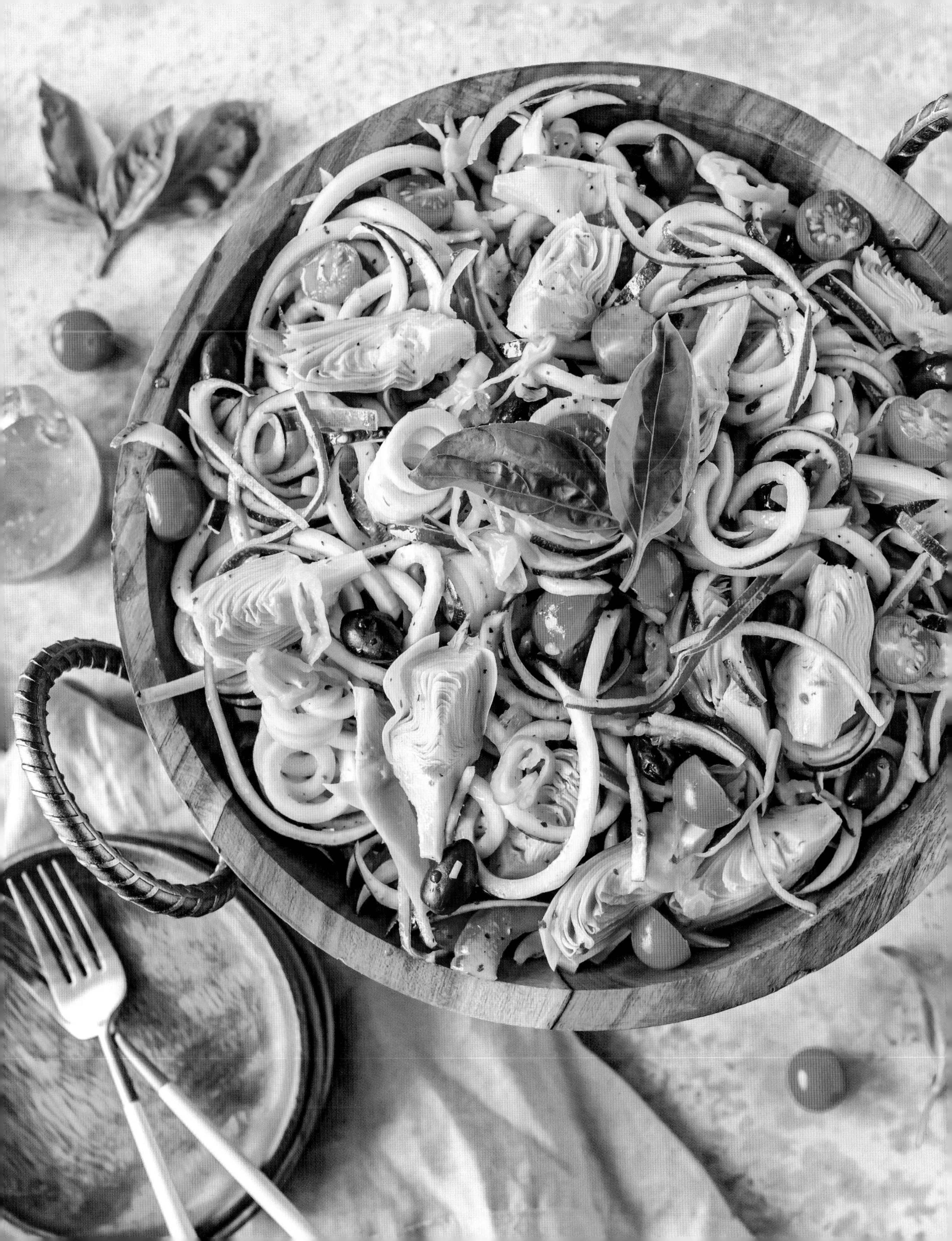

Balsamic Chicken over Tomato Salad

This tender balsamic chicken breast is served over a traditional tomato-cucumber salad and drizzled with ranch dressing for a bold salad that's everything except boring.

SQUEAKY CLEAN PALEO / KETO PALEO / TRADITIONAL PALEO

Makes: 5 servings / **Prep Time:** 10 minutes / **Total Time:** 45 minutes + marinating time

BALSAMIC MARINADE

½ cup (120 ml) balsamic vinegar
¼ cup (60 ml) compliant chicken broth
3 tablespoons (45 ml) olive oil, divided
2 cloves garlic, minced
1½ teaspoons ground mustard powder
¼ teaspoon onion powder
5 boneless, skinless chicken breasts (4 to 6 ounces [112 to 168 g] each)

TOMATO SALAD

3½ cups (525 g) halved grape tomatoes
3 mini cucumbers, sliced
½ cup (80 g) chopped red onion
1 small avocado, peeled, pitted, and cubed
2½ tablespoons (37 ml) light olive oil
Juice of ½ lemon
1½ tablespoons (23 ml) red wine vinegar
1 teaspoon dried oregano
½ teaspoon garlic powder
½ teaspoon dried parsley
½ teaspoon dried basil
½ teaspoon sea salt
½ teaspoon black pepper
Ranch Dressing (page 30) or compliant dressing of choice, for garnish
Fresh sliced basil, for garnish

BALSAMIC MARINADE

1. In a medium bowl, whisk together the vinegar, broth, 2 tablespoons (30 ml) of the olive oil, garlic, mustard, and onion powder.
2. Transfer to a gallon-size resealable plastic bag. Add the chicken and gently toss to coat with the marinade.
3. Marinate between 30 minutes and 1 hour. (For best flavor, marinate overnight in the refrigerator. Set the bag in a baking dish or plate.)
4. Grease the grill with the remaining 1 tablespoon (15 ml) olive oil and preheat to 400°F (200°C) or medium-high.
5. Place the chicken breasts on the grill and cook until the internal temperature reaches 160°F (71°C), 5 to 8 minutes per side, depending on the thickness of the breasts. Set aside.

TOMATO SALAD

1. In a large bowl, combine the tomatoes, cucumbers, onion, and avocado, gently mixing together with a spoon.
2. In a small bowl, whisk together the olive oil, lemon juice, vinegar, oregano, garlic powder, parsley, dried basil, salt, and pepper. Pour over the tomato salad and mix until well coated.
3. Divide the salad among 5 plates and top each with a chicken breast. Drizzle the breast with the ranch and garnish with fresh basil.

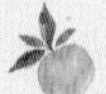

RECIPE NOTES

If you are not following Squeaky Clean or Keto Paleo, feel free to add 2 tablespoons (40 g) honey to the marinade.

BBQ Ranch Salad

I can eat BBQ anytime, anywhere. Sometimes I have to change up the way I serve it, and this BBQ Ranch Salad is simple yet flavorful. The salad includes *only* six ingredients and can be whipped up in a flash.

SQUEAKY CLEAN PALEO / KETO PALEO / TRADITIONAL PALEO

Makes: 4 servings / **Prep Time:** 5 minutes / **Total Time:** 15 minutes

- 8 slices pineapple, or ½ avocado if Keto
- 6 cups (360 g) kale salad mix
- 4 cups (560 g) cooked Shredded Pork, warmed (page 140)
- 1 cup (200 g) pickle slices, divided
- ½ red onion, sliced
- 1 cup (240 ml) Ranch Dressing (page 30) or compliant ranch dressing
- 2½ tablespoons (37 ml) BBQ Sauce (page 35) or compliant BBQ sauce

1. Place the pineapple slices on a grill or griddle and cook until tender and grill marks are visible on both sides, about 2 minutes per side. Cut into chunks.
2. Assemble the salad by adding 1½ cups (90 g) of the kale to each of 4 bowls or plates. Divide the pork, pineapple, pickles, and onion evenly among the salads.
3. Add the ranch and BBQ sauce to a wide-mouth mason jar or medium bowl and shake or stir to combine.
4. Drizzle the BBQ ranch over the salads before serving. Cap the remaining dressing in a jar and refrigerate for up to 1 week.

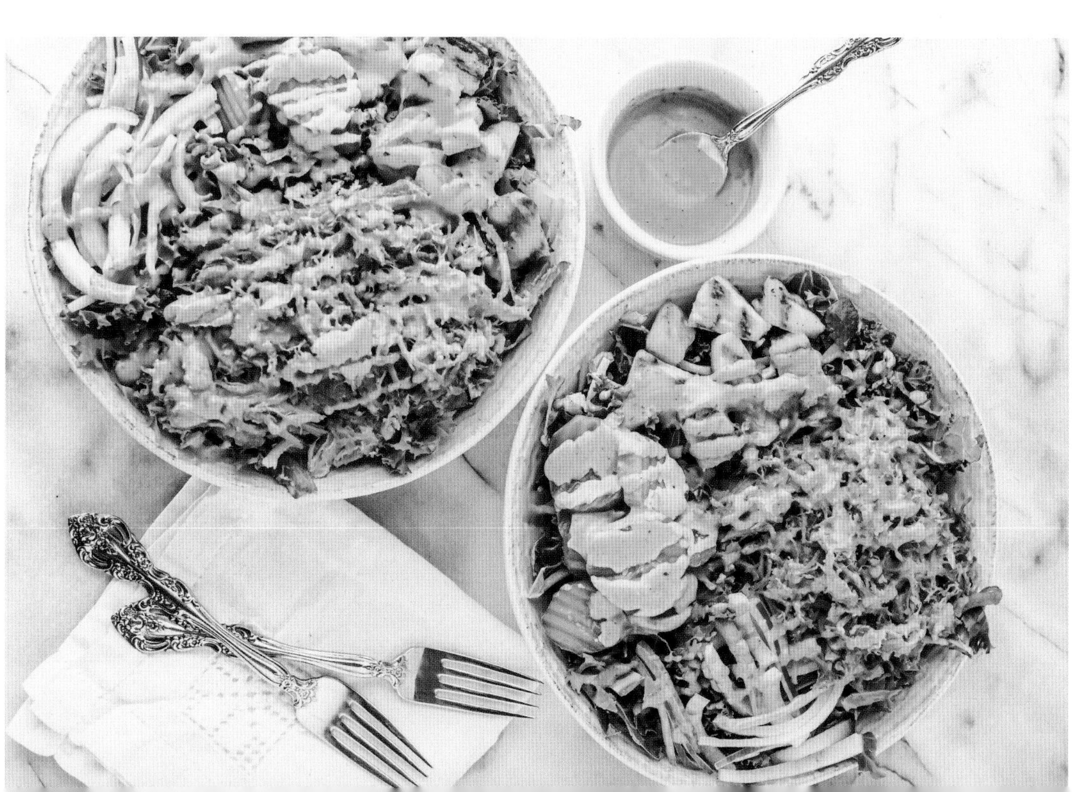

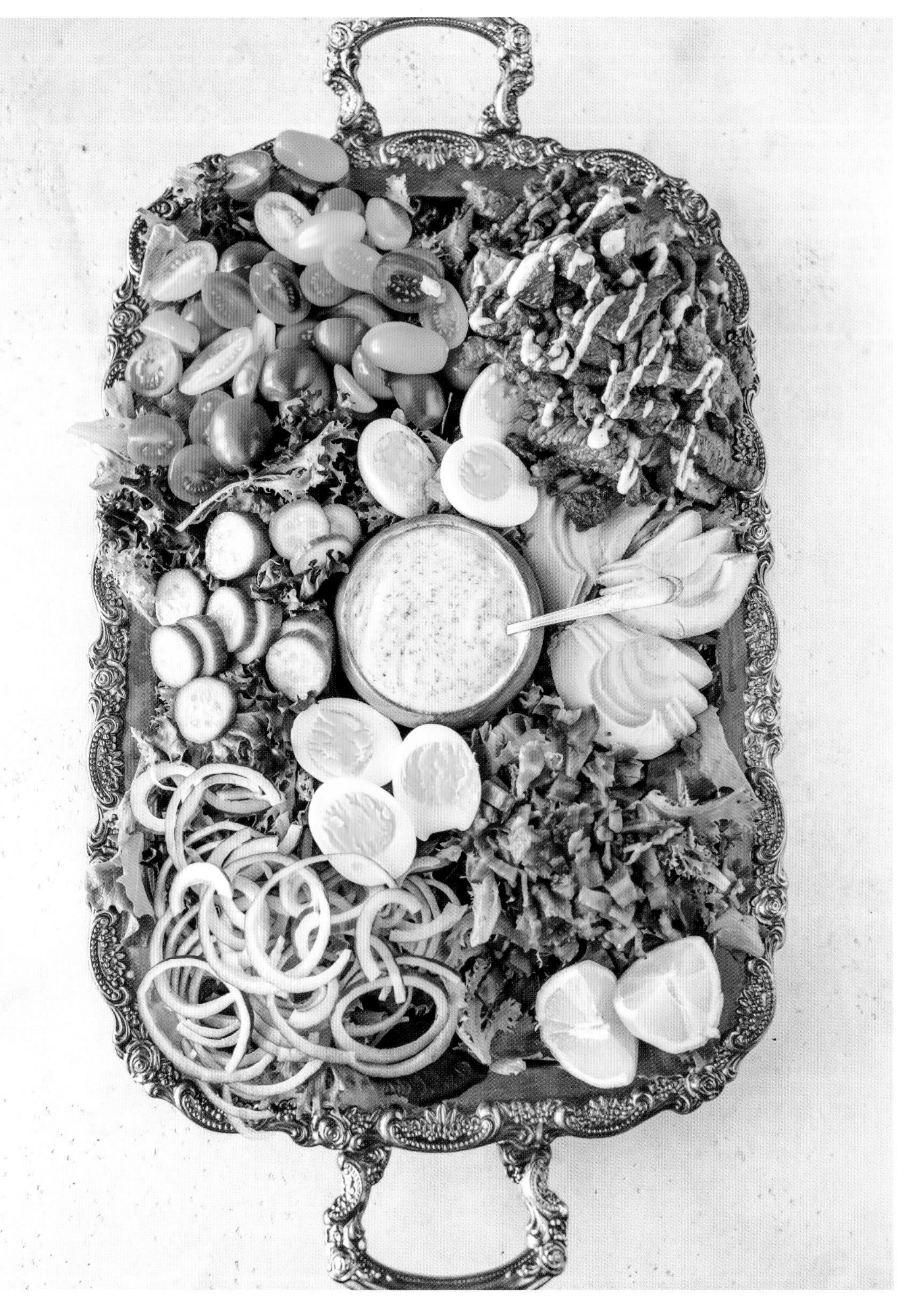

Cobb Steak Salad Platter

This simple and craveable steak cobb salad is filled with sirloin steak pieces, boiled eggs, red onion, crumbled bacon, sliced avocado, and cucumbers, and drizzled with homemade ranch.

SQUEAKY CLEAN PALEO / KETO PALEO / TRADITIONAL PALEO

Makes: 6 servings / **Prep Time:** 10 minutes / **Total Time:** 25 to 30 minutes

3 slices compliant bacon
3 large eggs
1 tablespoon (15 ml) olive oil
1½ pounds (680 g) flank steak
8 cups (240 g) lettuce mix of choice
1½ cups (225 g) halved multicolor grape tomatoes
½ red onion, sliced
2 mini cucumbers, sliced
1 large avocado, peeled, pitted, and sliced
1 cup Ranch Dressing (page 28)
1 lemon, cut into wedges, for garnish

1. Preheat the oven to 400°F (200°C or gas mark 6).
2. Place the bacon on a baking sheet. Bake until the desired doneness, 15 to 20 minutes.
3. Transfer the cooked bacon to a paper towel to drain excess oil. Chop when cool.
4. Meanwhile, place the eggs in a single layer in a saucepan and cover them with cool water. Heat over high heat until the water begins to boil, then cover with a lid and turn the heat to low. Cook for a minute or two, then remove the pan from the heat. Leave the eggs, covered, for an additional 13 minutes.
5. Prepare an ice bath by adding ice and water to a large bowl. Use a slotted spoon to transfer the boiled eggs to the ice water. Allow to sit for a couple of minutes, until cool enough to handle.
6. Peel the eggs and slice in half lengthwise. Set aside.
7. Heat the oil in a large skillet over medium-high heat.
8. Add the steak and cook until the desired doneness, 5 to 6 minutes. Thinly slice against the grain.
9. Place the lettuce mix on a big platter. Top with the tomatoes, onion, cucumbers, avocado, eggs, steak, and bacon.
10. Drizzle with the dressing and serve with lemon wedges.

Tuna Salad-Stuffed Avocados

Forget those tuna salads in a pouch. This dill pickle-infused version is just as creamy but is extra satisfying when stuffed into an avocado half. It can serve as the perfect lunch or snack throughout the week. Simply make the tuna salad early in the week and cut the avocados "to order."

SQUEAKY CLEAN PALEO / KETO PALEO / TRADITIONAL PALEO

Makes: 6 servings / **Prep Time:** 8 minutes / **Total Time:** 20 minutes

2 large eggs
4 cans (5 ounces [140 g]) tuna packed in water, drained
1 cup (240 g) Mayo (page 28) or compliant mayonnaise
3 no-sugar-added dill pickles, finely chopped
¼ cup (40 g) chopped red onion
1 tablespoon (15 ml) lemon juice
½ teaspoon sea salt, or to taste
¼ teaspoon black pepper, or to taste
¼ teaspoon garlic powder
3 medium avocados, halved and pitted (see Note)

1. Place the eggs in a small saucepan and cover with water. Heat on high heat until the water begins to boil, then cover with a lid and turn the heat to low. Cook for a minute or two. Remove from the heat, and leave the eggs covered an additional 13 minutes. Transfer to a bowl of ice water, then peel when cool enough to handle. Chop the eggs.
2. Add the tuna to a medium bowl.
3. Add the eggs, mayo, pickles, red onion, lemon juice, salt, pepper, and garlic powder. Mix until well combined.
4. Use a spoon to scoop out some of the avocado from the pitted areas to widen where the tuna salad will sit.
5. Divide the tuna salad and spoon it onto each half of the avocados.
6. Serve immediately or store the tuna salad only, covered, in the fridge for up to 4 days. (Don't cut the avocados until you're ready to use them.)

RECIPE NOTES

To pit an avocado, make a lengthwise cut, slicing until the blade hits the pit. Pick up the avocado and give it a twist. The two halves should come right apart. Pick up the half with the pit in it. Carefully hit the pit with the edge of a chef's knife until it sticks. Twist and lift out the pit.

Creamy Broccoli Salad with Apple

This crunchy salad is filled with broccoli and cauliflower florets, apples, and red onion. Drenched in ranch dressing and topped with crispy bacon, it's perfect for social gatherings, backyard picnics, or holiday events. What's even better is that you can make it the day before and just take it out when it's time to eat.

SQUEAKY CLEAN PALEO / TRADITIONAL PALEO

Makes: 6 servings / **Prep Time:** 10 minutes / **Total Time:** 25 minutes

3 pieces compliant bacon
3 cups (210 g) broccoli florets
3 cups (300 g) cauliflower florets
1 cup (150 g) cubed red apple, skin on
1 small red onion, finely chopped
1 cup (240 ml) Ranch Dressing (page 30)
3 tablespoons (18 g) chopped scallion
Sea salt and black pepper, to taste

1. Preheat the oven to 400°F (200°C or gas mark 6).
2. Place the bacon on a baking sheet and bake until the desired doneness, 15 to 20 minutes.
3. Transfer the cooked bacon to a paper towel to drain excess oil. Chop when cool.
4. Meanwhile, in a large bowl, combine the broccoli, cauliflower, apple, and onion.
5. Add the ranch and mix with a wooden spoon until everything is well combined.
6. Sprinkle the bacon and scallion over the top of the salad.
7. Serve immediately for best results.

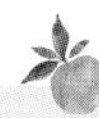

RECIPE NOTES

To make this side dish Keto Paleo, simply remove the apples.

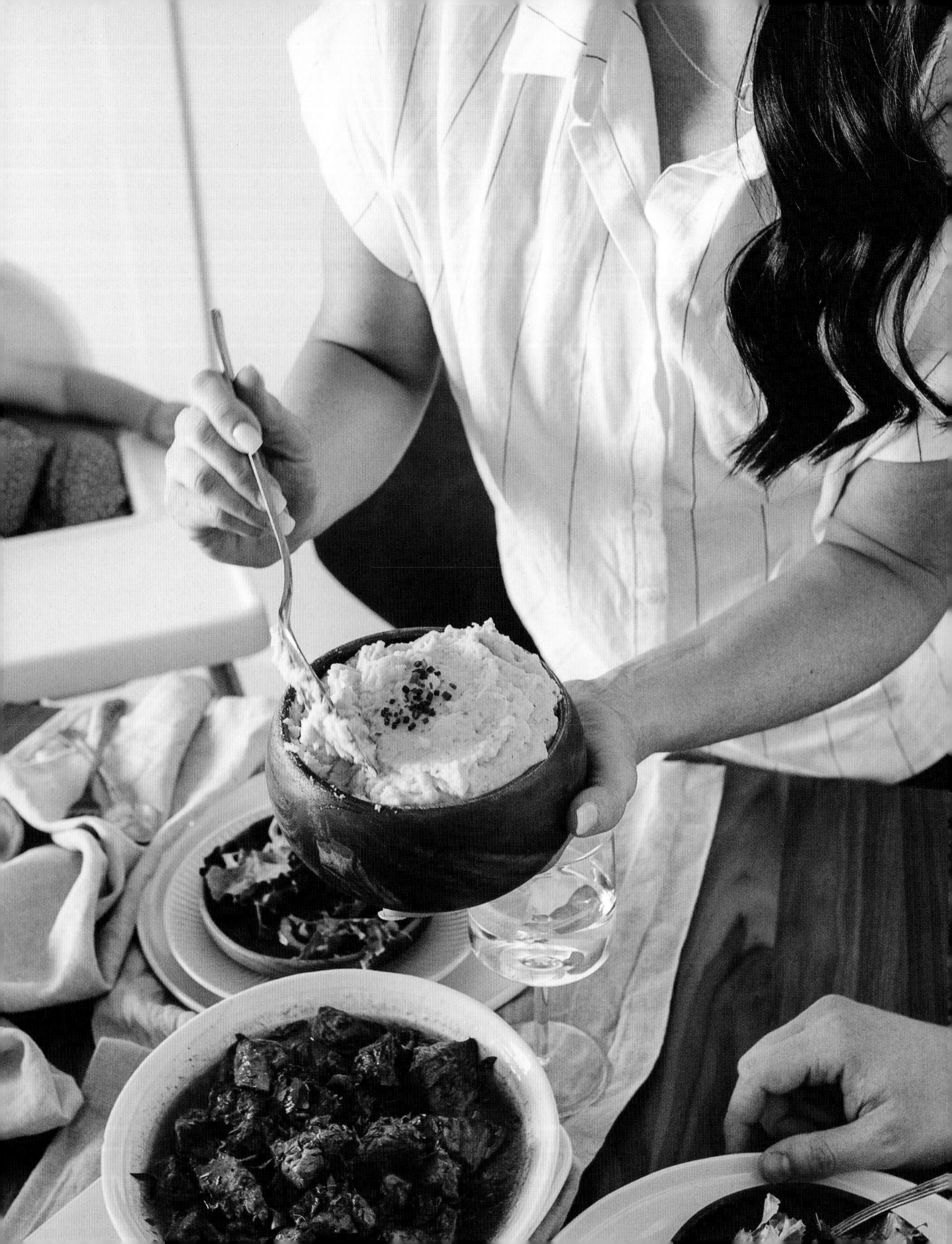

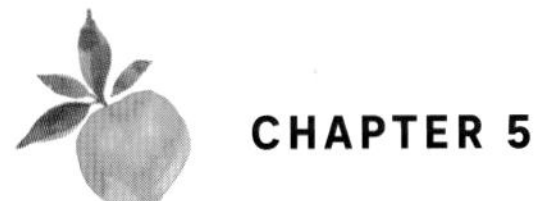

CHAPTER 5

Side Dishes

I grew up with a momma who made ten side dishes to go with every meal. I know that's a little extreme, but I think it's why I have a deep love for my sides. Sometimes, if you have a boring protein option, a great way to brighten up your meal is with a delicious side dish, like my Creamy Brussels Sprouts (page 90) or Asian Green Beans and Mushrooms (page 91).

Sue Sue's Creamy Baked Tomatoes

My Grandmother Sue Sue's beloved creamy baked tomato recipe is not only out-of-this-world delicious, but it also holds such a special place in my heart and tummy. My hopes are that this recipe will bring lots of love into your home, just as it has mine.

SQUEAKY CLEAN PALEO / KETO PALEO / TRADITIONAL PALEO

Makes: 12 tomato slices / **Prep Time:** 5 minutes / **Total Time:** 15 minutes

3 large beefsteak tomatoes, sliced ¼ inch (6 mm) thick

¾ cup (180 ml) Mac's Awesome Sauce (page 31)

Fresh chopped basil, for garnish

1. Preheat the oven to 400°F (200°C or gas mark 6). Line a baking sheet with parchment paper.
2. Place the tomatoes on the prepared baking sheet. Top each tomato with 1 tablespoon (15 ml) of the Awesome Sauce. Bake for 10 minutes.
3. Turn the oven to broil. Broil for 2 to 3 minutes to brown the top of the sauce. Be careful not to burn the top. Keep a close eye during this step.
4. Remove from the oven and sprinkle the top of each tomato with the basil. Serve immediately.

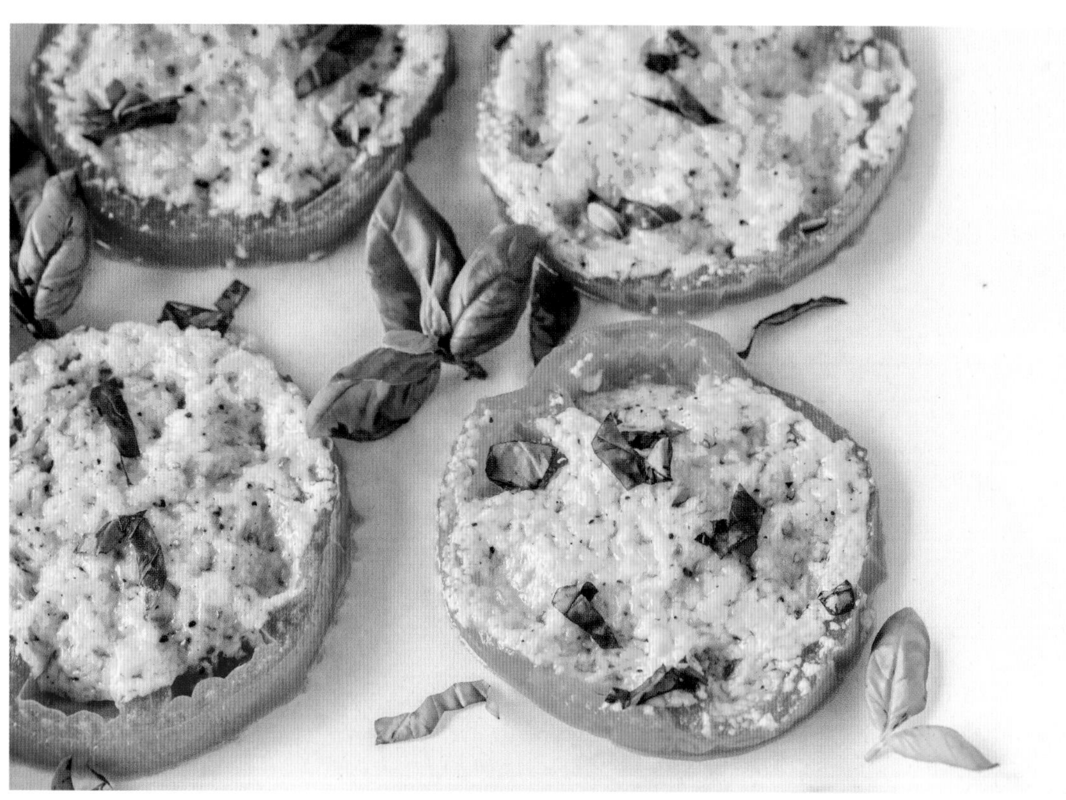

Mexican Cauliflower Rice

This super-easy, Mexican-inspired cauliflower rice is a must for your next Taco Tuesday. It's infused with amazing Mexican flavors, such as paprika, cumin, jalapeño, and cilantro.

SQUEAKY CLEAN PALEO / KETO PALEO / TRADITIONAL PALEO

Makes: 4 servings / **Prep Time:** 5 minutes / **Total Time:** 15 minutes

1 large head cauliflower, trimmed and cut into florets (see Note)
1 tablespoon (15 ml) olive oil
½ medium yellow onion, diced
1 jalapeño, seeded and sliced (optional)
2 cloves garlic, minced
⅓ cup (80 ml) compliant beef broth
3½ tablespoons (52 g) tomato paste
Juice of ½ lime
1 teaspoon ground cumin
½ teaspoon paprika
Sea salt and black pepper to taste
Chopped cilantro, for garnish

1. Add the cauliflower florets to a food processor. Pulse until the cauliflower resembles small rice-like bits. Make sure not to overpulse.
2. Heat the olive oil in a large skillet over medium heat, then add the onion, jalapeño (if using), and garlic.
3. Add the riced cauliflower and cook until tender, about 4 minutes.
4. In a separate bowl, whisk together the broth, tomato paste, and lime juice. Pour into the skillet and stir to combine.
5. Season with the cumin, paprika, and a pinch of salt and pepper. Taste and add more salt and pepper, if necessary.
6. Garnish with the cilantro before serving.

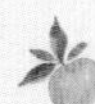

RECIPE NOTES

You can buy cauliflower rice pretty much everywhere these days (though it's expensive!). If you go that route, use about 5 cups (700 g) for this recipe.

Creamy Brussels Sprouts

If you haven't been a fan of Brussels sprouts before, you're in for a surprise. And if you do like them, well, you're in for a real treat. Here, I add flavor to plain sprouts by cooking them in a cream sauce and topping with crumbled bacon. You'll want to keep this dish all to yourself.

SQUEAKY CLEAN PALEO / KETO PALEO / TRADITIONAL PALEO

Makes: 5 or 6 servings / **Prep Time:** 5 minutes / **Total Time:** 15 minutes

- 3 slices compliant bacon
- 1½ tablespoons (23 ml) olive oil
- 2 small shallots, diced
- 2 cloves garlic, minced
- 2 pounds (910 g) Brussels sprouts, trimmed and halved
- 1 cup (240 ml) canned unsweetened coconut milk
- ¼ cup (60 ml) no sugar added beef broth
- 1 tablespoon (4 g) nutritional yeast
- 1 teaspoon crushed red pepper flakes
- Sea salt and black pepper, to taste
- 1½ teaspoons tapioca flour or arrowroot powder, dissolved in 2 teaspoons water (see Note)

1. Preheat the oven to 400°F (200°C or gas mark 6).
2. Place the bacon on a baking sheet. Bake until the desired doneness, 15 to 20 minutes.
3. Transfer the cooked bacon to a paper towel to drain the excess oil. Chop when cool.
4. Meanwhile, heat the olive oil in a large skillet over medium-high heat. Add the shallots and garlic and cook, stirring frequently, until fragrant and tender, 1 to 2 minutes.
5. Add the Brussels sprouts. Cook, stirring occasionally, until tender, 8 to 10 minutes.
6. Add the coconut milk, broth, nutritional yeast, red pepper flakes, and a generous pinch of salt and pepper. Stir together with a spoon until all the ingredients are combined.
7. Add the tapioca mixture. Turn the heat to low and cook until the sauce thickens, 4 to 5 minutes more.
8. Crumble the bacon over the top of the Brussels sprouts before serving.

RECIPE NOTES

For a Keto Paleo thickening agent, subsitute 1½ tablespoons (14 g) gelatin or ¼ teaspoon xanthan gum for the tapioca flour.

Asian Green Beans and Mushrooms

Green beans and mushrooms are the new peas and carrots. When cooked in coconut aminos, rice vinegar, sesame oil, ginger, and garlic, they're perfect to serve with chicken or a Paleo-inspired main dish.

SQUEAKY CLEAN PALEO / KETO PALEO / TRADITIONAL PALEO

Makes: 4 servings / **Prep Time:** 3 minutes / **Total Time:** 15 minutes

1 pound (454 g) fresh green beans, trimmed
1 tablespoon (14 g) ghee
2 cloves garlic, minced
1½ cups (105 g) button mushrooms
¼ cup (60 ml) coconut aminos
1 tablespoon (15 ml) sesame oil
1 tablespoon (15 ml) rice vinegar
¼ teaspoon ground ginger
Sesame seeds, for garnish

1. Prepare a large bowl of ice and water.
2. Bring a pot of water to a boil and blanch the green beans until they are bright green, about 2 minutes. Immediately transfer the green beans to the ice water.
3. Once the green beans are cool, drain and pat dry using a dish towel.
4. Heat the ghee in a large skillet over medium heat until the ghee sizzles. Add the garlic and stir for about 30 seconds.
5. Add the mushrooms and cook until tender, 2 to 3 minutes.
6. Transfer the green beans to the skillet and toss together. Cook for 5 minutes.
7. In a small bowl, whisk together the coconut aminos, sesame oil, vinegar, and ginger.
8. Reduce the heat to low and add the liquid mixture to the skillet. Stir well and simmer for 1 to 2 minutes more.
9. Sprinkle with the sesame seeds and serve immediately.

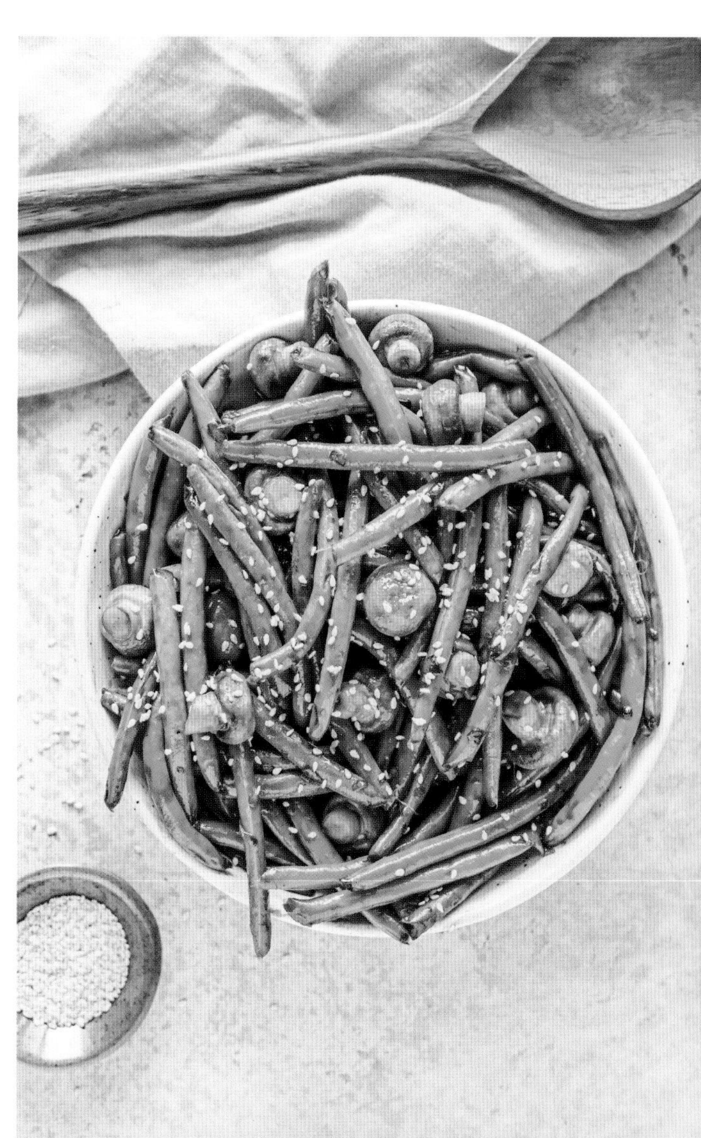

Smashed Sweet Potato Slices

These smashed sweet potatoes are baked until tender and then drizzled with a garlic-ghee sauce. They're great served on salads, or even alongside a protein. Get creative by adding shredded pork or chicken over the top.

SQUEAKY CLEAN PALEO / TRADITIONAL PALEO

Makes: 4 servings / **Prep Time:** 10 minutes / **Total Time:** 30 to 35 minutes

3 large sweet potatoes, sliced into 1-inch (2.5 cm)-thick rounds
¼ cup (60 ml) melted ghee
2½ teaspoons dried parsley
1 teaspoon sea salt, divided
½ teaspoon garlic powder
Black pepper, to taste
Chopped fresh parsley, for garnish (optional)

1. Preheat the oven to 425°F (220°C or gas mark 7). Coat a baking sheet with olive oil cooking spray.
2. Transfer the sweet potatoes to the prepared baking sheet. Bake until the potatoes are fork tender, 25 to 30 minutes.
3. Take a fork and press each sweet potato slice down until flattened.
4. In a small bowl, combine the ghee, parsley, ½ teaspoon of the salt, and garlic powder.
5. Pour the ghee mixture over each potato round.
6. Sprinkle each round with the remaining ½ teaspoon salt and pepper to taste.
7. Garnish with fresh parsley, if desired, before serving.

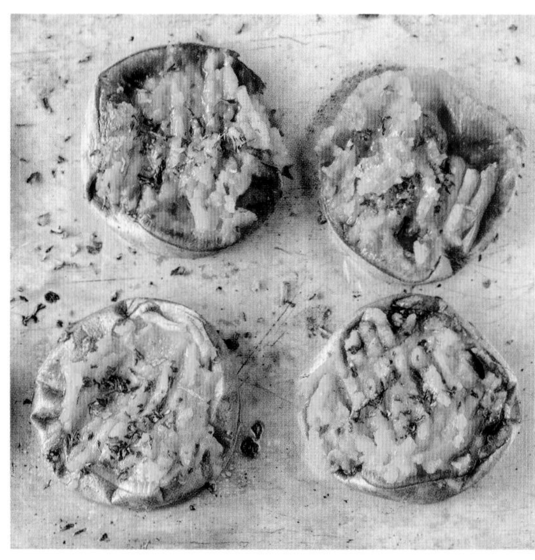

Cajun Parsnip Fries with Fry Sauce

Enough with the sweet potato fries! These parsnip fries are a game changer and will break your boring sweet potato fry streak. Dip in Boom Boom Fry Sauce (page 53) and devour!

SQUEAKY CLEAN PALEO / TRADITIONAL PALEO

Makes: 4 servings / **Prep Time:** 10 minutes / **Total Time:** 30 minutes

6 parsnips, peeled, ends trimmed
1 tablespoon (6 g) paprika
1 teaspoon dried thyme
1 teaspoon dried oregano
1 teaspoon garlic powder
1 teaspoon sea salt
1 teaspoon black pepper
½ teaspoon onion powder
¼ teaspoon cayenne pepper
2 tablespoons (30 ml) olive oil
Boom Boom Fry Sauce (page 53)

1. Preheat the oven to 400°F (200°C or gas mark 6). Line a baking sheet with parchment paper.
2. Cut the parsnips into fries, 3 inches (7.5 cm) long and ½ inch (1.3 cm) thick. Add them to a large mixing bowl.
3. In a small bowl, whisk together the paprika, thyme, oregano, garlic powder, salt, black pepper, onion powder, and cayenne pepper.
4. Add the olive oil to the parsnips. Mix together until the fries are evenly coated.
5. Sprinkle the seasoning over the fries. Toss with your hands to ensure they are evenly coated. Transfer to the prepared baking sheet.
6. Bake until golden brown, flipping halfway through, 20 to 25 minutes.
7. Serve with the Boom Boom Fry Sauce.

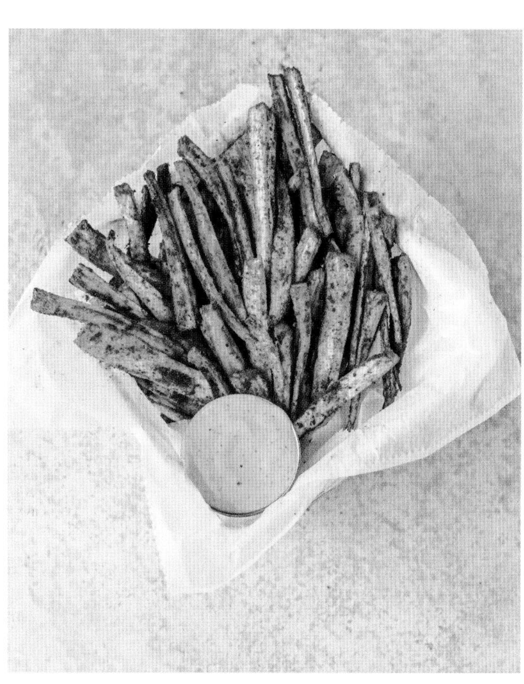

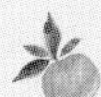

RECIPE NOTES

Cook time will depend on your oven. Keep a close eye to ensure the fries don't burn. Adjust the time accordingly. If you don't like parsnips, use 2 large sweet potatoes instead.

Roasted Cabbage Steaks with Garlic Aioli and Bacon

These roasted cabbage steaks are a garlic lover's dream. Drizzled with fresh garlic aioli and crumbled crispy bacon, they're a great accompaniment to steak—but they're hearty enough on their own.

SQUEAKY CLEAN PALEO / KETO PALEO / TRADITIONAL PALEO

Makes: 5 or 6 servings / **Prep Time:** 10 minutes / **Total Time:** 35 to 40 minutes

---

1 head green cabbage
2½ tablespoons (37 ml) olive oil
Sea salt and black pepper, to taste
3 slices compliant bacon

GARLIC AIOLI

1 cup (240 g) Mayo (page 28) or compliant mayonnaise
2 cloves garlic
1 teaspoon Dijon mustard
Sea salt, to taste
¼ teaspoon black pepper

---

1. Preheat the oven to 400°F (200°C or gas mark 6). Oil a baking sheet.
2. Slice the cabbage vertically into ½-inch (1.3 cm)-thick steaks (you should get 5 or 6 slices).
3. Place the cabbage steaks on the prepared baking sheet and brush each steak with the olive oil. Sprinkle with salt and pepper.
4. Bake until the cabbage is tender and the edges are browned and a little crispy, 30 to 35 minutes.
5. Meanwhile, place the bacon on a separate baking sheet. Bake until the desired doneness, 15 to 20 minutes. Transfer the cooked bacon to a paper towel to drain excess oil, then place on a cutting board and chop.
6. Remove the cabbage from the oven and transfer the cabbage steaks to a serving platter.
7. To serve, drizzle with the aioli and top with the bacon.

GARLIC AIOLI

Put the mayo, garlic, mustard, salt, and pepper in a wide-mouth mason jar and blend together using an immersion blender. Taste and add more salt and pepper, if necessary. (You can also make this in a regular blender.)

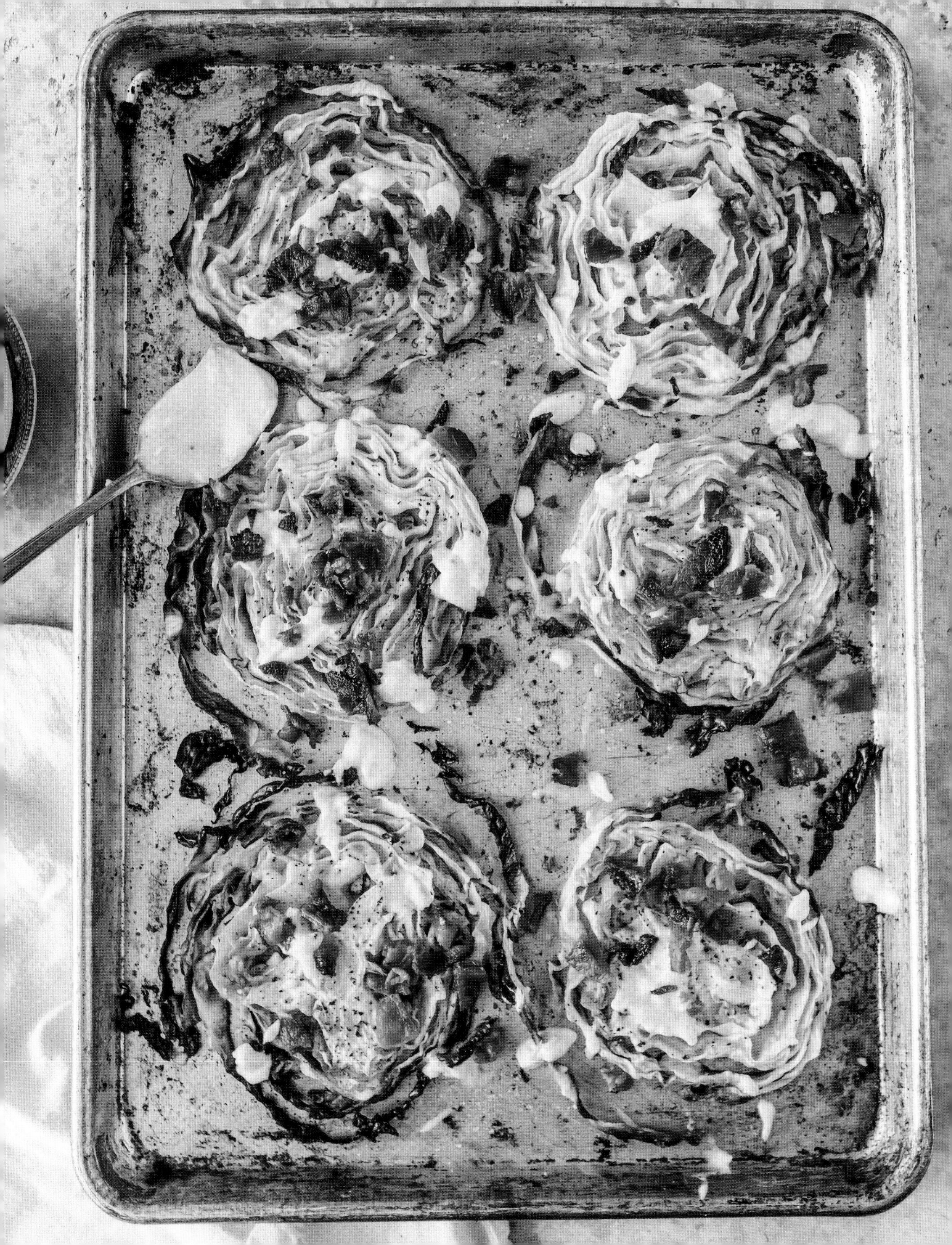

Cauliflower Mash

All hail the cauliflower mash! So simple, yet so delicious. Did I mention it tastes better than mashed potatoes? It's amazing covered in Pot Roast (page 144), Beef Tips (page 140), or served as a side for pork chops, steak, or chicken.

SQUEAKY CLEAN PALEO / KETO PALEO / TRADITIONAL PALEO

Makes: 4 servings / **Prep Time:** 5 minutes / **Total Time:** 15 minutes

2 bags (12 ounces [336 g]) frozen cauliflower florets or 1 head cauliflower, trimmed and chopped (see Note)
2 tablespoons (30 ml) canned unsweetened coconut milk
1 tablespoon (1 g) chopped fresh chives, plus more for garnish
2 teaspoons ghee
¾ teaspoon sea salt
½ teaspoon garlic powder
1 teaspoon black pepper

1. In a large pot of water, bring the cauliflower to a boil over high heat until tender, about 8 minutes.
2. Drain and transfer the cauliflower to a food processor or high-speed blender, along with the coconut milk, chives, ghee, salt, garlic powder, and pepper.
3. Blend until smooth. Make sure not to overblend or it will turn into a soupy puree. You want it to be mashed-potato consistency. If needed, add more coconut milk. Taste and add more salt, if desired.
4. Top with more chives before serving.

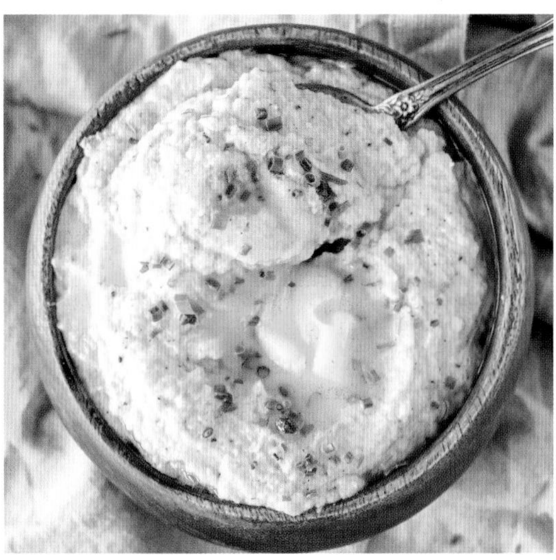

RECIPE NOTES

If you are using a head of cauliflower, add the florets to a food processor and pulse until it becomes a rice-like consistency. Add the rice to a microwave-safe bowl with 2 tablespoons (30 ml) water and microwave on high for 5 minutes. This will help make it tender and quicker to cook in step 1. You should get about 5 cups (700 g).

Roasted Asparagus and Tomatoes with Lemon Vinaigrette

Plain roasted asparagus isn't that appetizing. However, this roasted asparagus with tomatoes, drizzled with a creamy lemon vinaigrette and topped with crunchy macadamia nuts, is both appetizing and delicious. This is a great side to serve with any protein, especially steak.

SQUEAKY CLEAN PALEO / KETO PALEO / TRADITIONAL PALEO

Makes: 4 servings / **Prep Time:** 5 minutes / **Total Time:** 20 minutes

ASPARAGUS AND TOMATOES

1 bunch asparagus, ends trimmed
1½ cups (225 g) cherry tomatoes, halved
1½ tablespoons (23 ml) olive oil
¼ teaspoon sea salt
2 to 3 tablespoons (16 to 24 g) chopped macadamia nuts

LEMON VINAIGRETTE

3 tablespoons (45 ml) light olive oil
Juice of ½ lemon
½ teaspoon Dijon mustard
¼ teaspoon onion powder
⅛ teaspoon sea salt
Pinch of black pepper

ASPARAGUS AND TOMATOES

1. Preheat the oven to 400°F (200°C or gas mark 6) and coat a baking sheet with olive oil cooking spray.
2. Arrange the asparagus on one end of the baking sheet and the tomatoes on the other. Drizzle with the olive oil and sprinkle with the salt.
3. Bake until the veggies soften and start to brown, 15 to 20 minutes.
4. Remove the sheet pan from the oven and place the asparagus and tomatoes on a large plate. Top with the lemon vinaigrette and macadamia nuts.

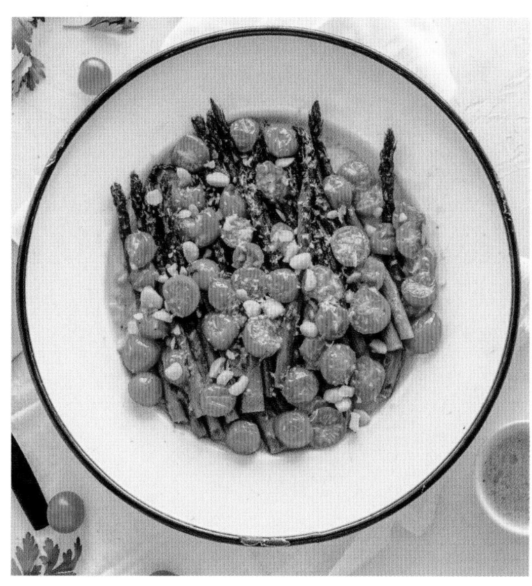

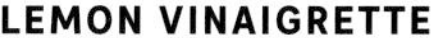

LEMON VINAIGRETTE

In a small bowl, whisk together the olive oil, lemon juice, mustard, onion powder, salt, and pepper.

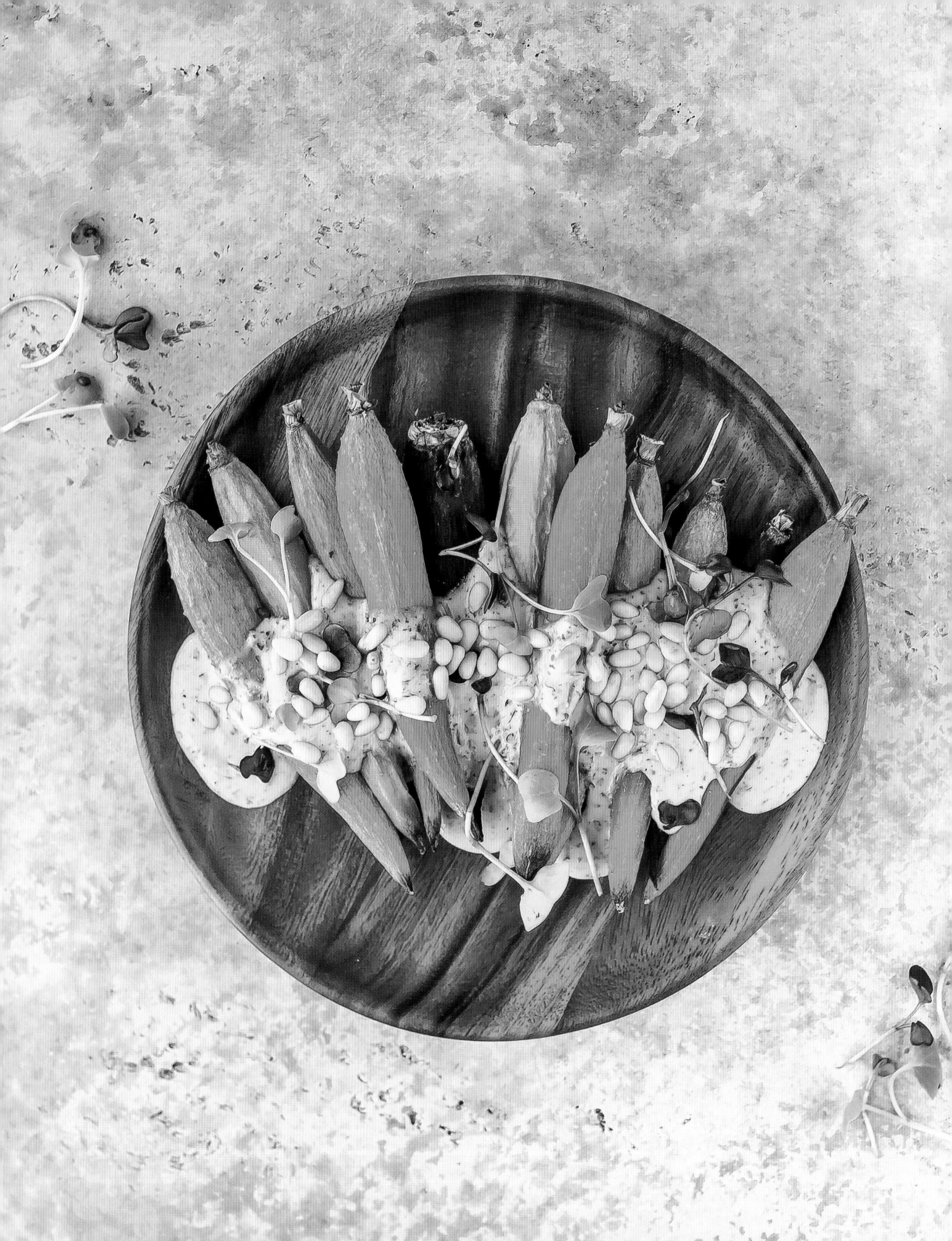

Roasted Carrots with Herb Tahini Dressing

These pretty roasted carrots, drizzled with an herbed tahini sauce, are the perfect side to chicken, pork, or steak.

SQUEAKY CLEAN PALEO / TRADITIONAL PALEO

Makes: 4 servings / **Prep Time:** 5 minutes / **Total Time:** 20 minutes

ROASTED CARROTS

1 large bunch rainbow carrots, scrubbed
1 tablespoon (15 ml) olive oil
½ teaspoon sea salt
2 tablespoons (16 g) pine nuts
Microgreens, for garnish (optional)

HERB TAHINI DRESSING

¼ cup (60 ml) extra-light olive oil
¼ cup (60 g) tahini
¼ cup (60 ml) water
Juice of 1 lemon
¼ cup (16 g) chopped fresh parsley
¼ cup (10 g) chopped fresh basil
2 tablespoons (6 g) chopped chives
1 clove garlic
Sea salt and black pepper, to taste

ROASTED CARROTS

1. Preheat the oven to 425°F (220°C or gas mark 7). Oil a baking sheet.
2. Place the carrots on the baking sheet. Drizzle with the olive oil and sprinkle with the salt. Toss to coat the carrots.
3. Roast until the carrots are tender and golden, about 20 minutes.
4. Remove the carrots from the oven and transfer to a plate.
5. Drizzle with 2 to 3 tablespoons (30 to 45 ml) of the Herb Tahini Dressing and sprinkle with the pine nuts. Garnish with microgreens, if desired.

HERB TAHINI DRESSING

1. Add the olive oil, tahini, water, lemon juice, parsley, basil, chives, garlic, and a pinch of salt and pepper to a high-speed blender or food processor. Blend until smooth, about 1 minute.
2. If the mixture is too thick, add a little more water. Taste and add more salt and pepper, if necessary.
3. Add any extra dressing to a mason jar and cap it with a lid. Will keep for up to 1 week in the fridge.

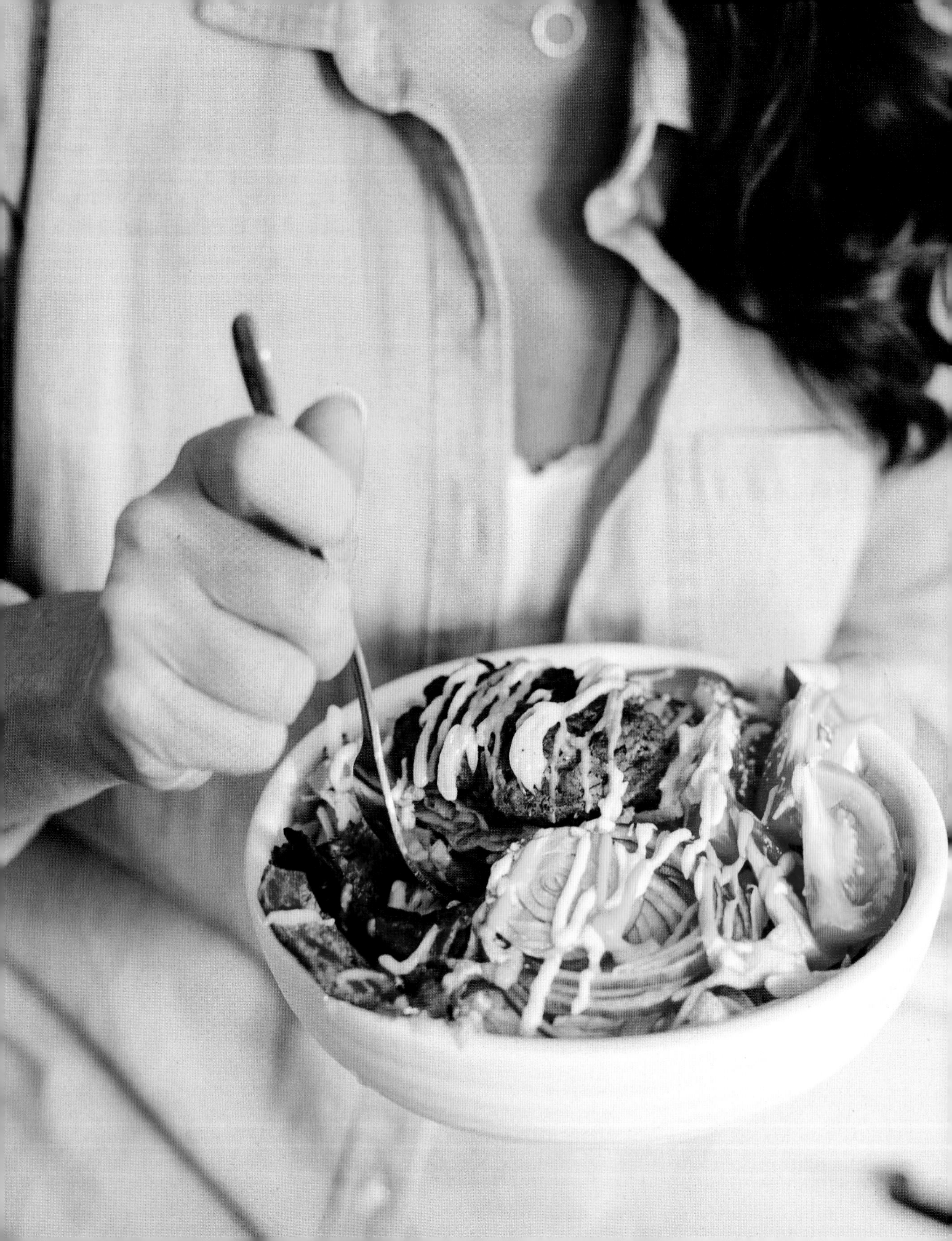

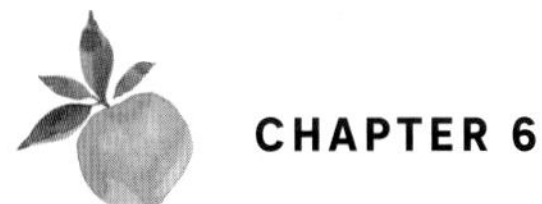

CHAPTER 6

Main Dishes

I am especially passionate about a main dish because it's the heart and soul of a meal. I vividly remember the dinners my momma would cook and serve our family. I still recall how her food made my tummy and heart feel, and I can still taste and smell her yummy beef stroganoff cooking in the kitchen. Food has a great way of pulling you back to a certain time and place in your life. My main dish recipes are made just for that: making memories and bringing the family together for a great meal and conversation around the kitchen table.

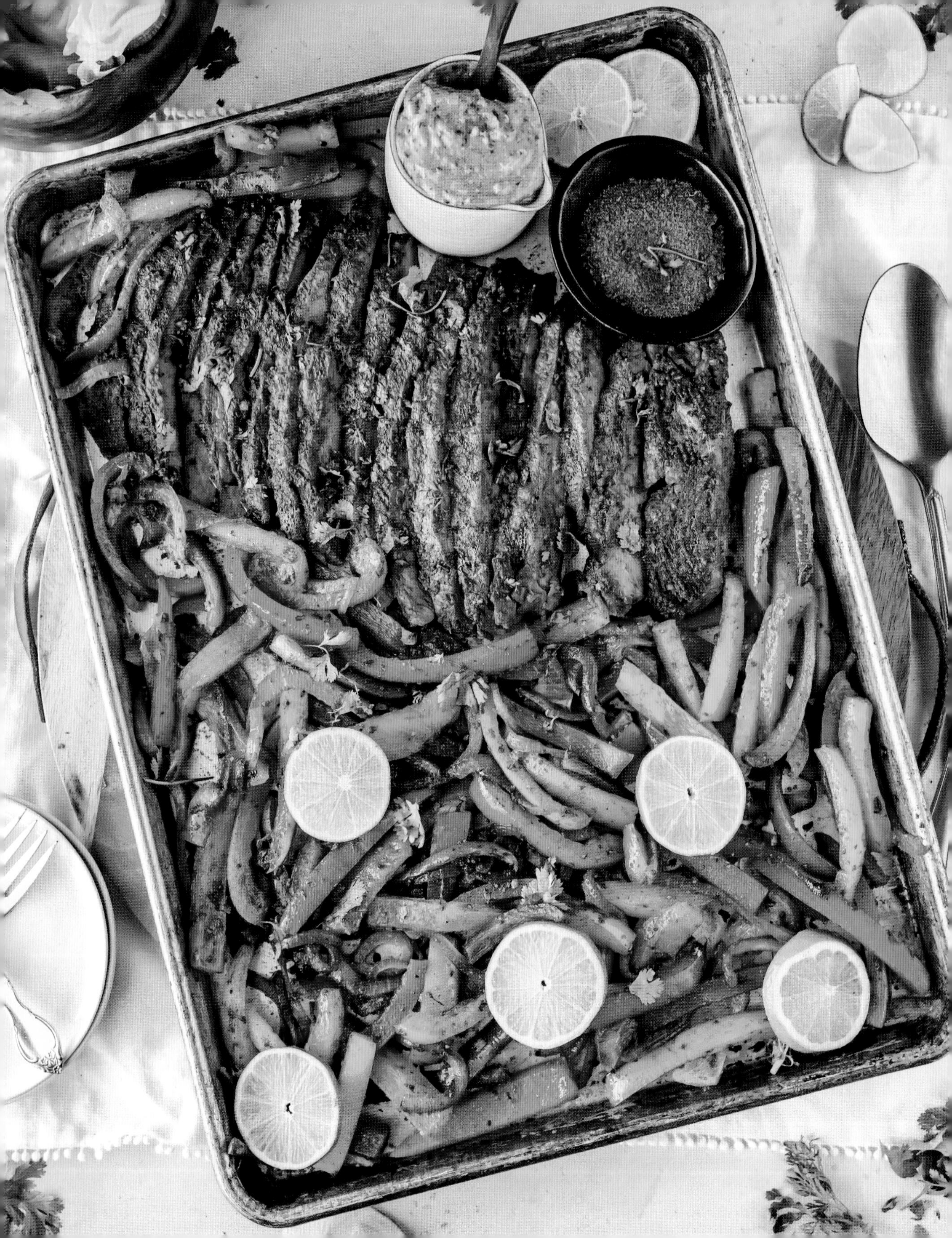

Sheet Pan Steak Fajitas

Sheet pan meals can be put together in no time and leave cleanup a piece of cake. Here, I stuff the tender steak fajita and veggies into a lettuce cup and top with a creamy avocado sauce for the perfect Paleo meal.

SQUEAKY CLEAN PALEO / KETO PALEO / TRADITIONAL PALEO

Makes: 4 servings / **Prep Time:** 10 minutes / **Total Time:** 25 to 30 minutes

Juice of 1 lime
1 tablespoon (15 ml) olive oil
2 teaspoons chili powder
1½ teaspoons garlic powder
1½ teaspoons dried oregano
1¼ teaspoons ground cumin
1 teaspoon paprika
1 teaspoon sea salt
1 teaspoon dried parsley
¼ teaspoon onion powder
¼ teaspoon black pepper
2 pounds (910 g) flank steak
1 red onion, sliced
1 red bell pepper, seeded and sliced
1 green bell pepper, seeded and sliced
1 orange bell pepper, seeded and sliced
8 to 12 butter lettuce leaves
Avocado Cilantro Cream (page 38)
Chopped cilantro, for garnish (optional)

1. Preheat the oven to 425°F (220°C or gas mark 7). Coat a rimmed baking sheet with olive oil cooking spray or olive oil.
2. In a small bowl, combine the lime juice and olive oil.
3. In a separate small bowl, whisk together the chili powder, garlic powder, oregano, cumin, paprika, salt, parsley, onion powder, and black pepper.
4. Set the steak on a cutting board and coat with half the lime juice mixture. Sprinkle half the seasoning all over the steak, top and bottom, and put on one end of the baking sheet.
5. Add the onion and bell peppers to a large bowl and toss with the remaining lime juice mixture and remaining spice blend. Scatter on the other end of the baking sheet, spreading them out so the full pan is covered.
6. Bake until the steak reaches your desired doneness, 12 to 15 minutes.
7. Remove the steak from the baking sheet to a cutting board to rest and return the vegetables to the oven until are tender, 5 minutes more.
8. After the steak has rested for 5 minutes, cut against the grain into ½-inch (1.3 cm) slices. Return to the baking sheet, if desired, to present the whole dish.
9. Serve the fajita steak and veggies in lettuce cups with Avocado Cilantro Cream drizzled on top and garnished with cilantro, if desired.

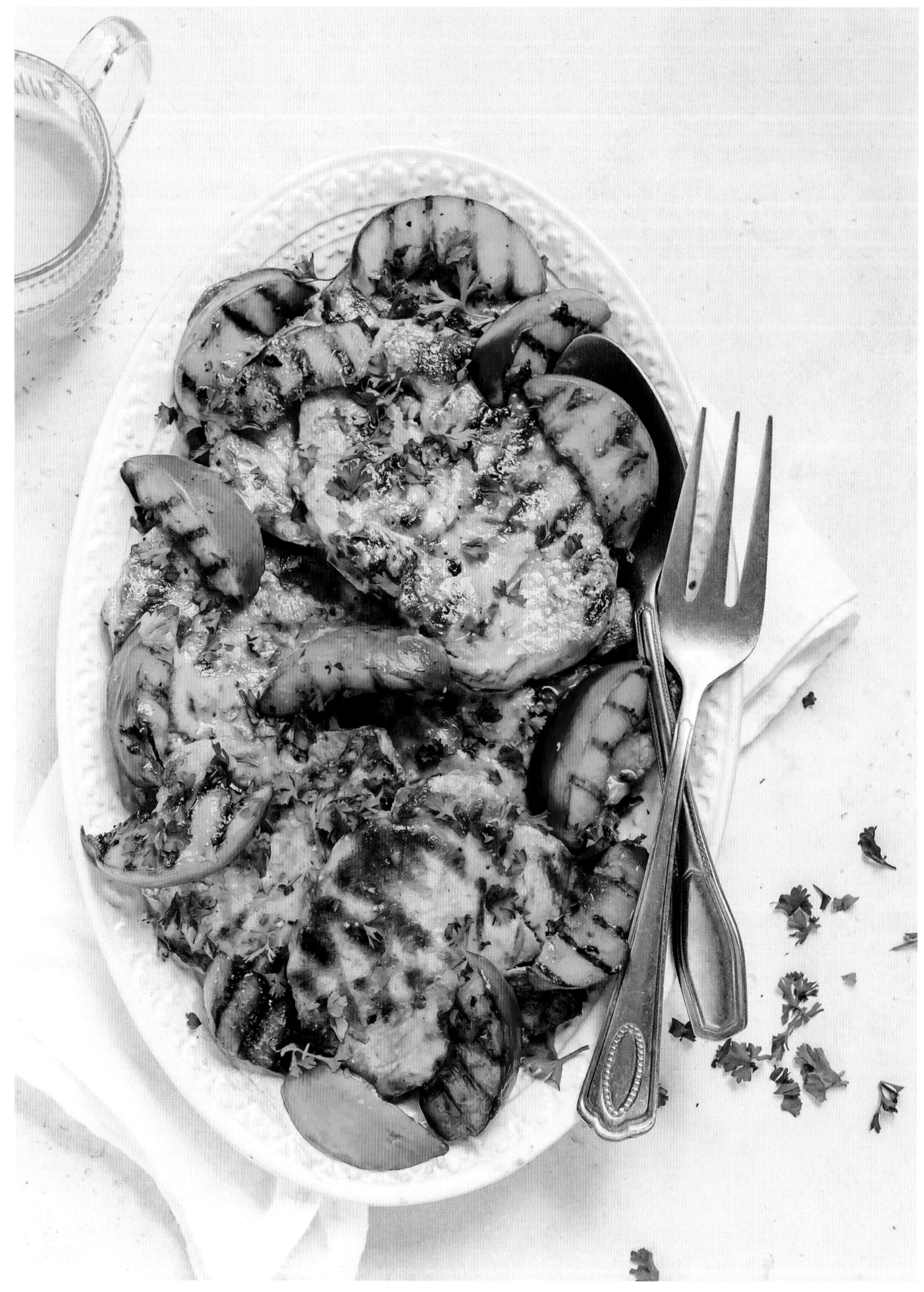

Grilled Pork Chops with Peach Vinaigrette

Pork chops don't have to be boring. These peach-inspired pork chops are both savory and sweet. To make this meal complete, serve with Cauliflower Mash (page 96) and green beans.

SQUEAKY CLEAN PALEO / TRADITIONAL PALEO

Makes: 6 servings / **Prep Time:** 7 minutes / **Total Time:** 20 minutes

6 bone-in pork chops (6 ounces [168 g] each)
1 cup (240 ml) Peach Vinaigrette (page 36)
2 large peaches, pitted and sliced
6 cups (180 g) arugula and spinach mix
Chopped fresh parsley, for garnish
Salt and pepper, to taste

1. Grease the grill and preheat to 400°F (200°C) or medium-high heat.
2. Place the pork chops on the grill and cook to your liking, 3 to 4 minutes on each side, depending on the thickness of the pork chop.
3. Transfer the pork chops to a platter and drizzle with the vinaigrette. Make sure to reserve a little bit of dressing to drizzle over the lettuce.
4. Grease the grill again and add the peaches. Cook until tender and grill marks have appeared, 2 to 3 minutes on each side.
5. To serve, set a pork chop on each plate. Place 1 cup (30 g) of the arugula and spinach mix alongside the chop and top it with a few grilled peaches, a drizzle of the vinaigrette, and a sprinkle of parsley.

Shrimp Fried Rice with Bang Bang Sauce

This shrimp fried rice is a great fakeout takeout meal. Even though it's a healthy spin on the traditional recipe, you would never know it. The flavors are spot-on and it's a perfect addition to a cozy Friday night.

SQUEAKY CLEAN PALEO / KETO PALEO / TRADITIONAL PALEO

Makes: 4 to 5 servings / **Prep Time:** 5 minutes / **Total Time:** 20 minutes

1½ tablespoons (23 ml) sesame oil, divided
1 pound (454 g) large peeled and deveined shrimp
2 large eggs
1 cup (100 g) chopped green beans
⅓ cup (40 g) chopped carrots
1 small shallot, diced
¼ cup (25 g) chopped scallions, plus more for garnish
2 cloves garlic, minced
6 cups (840 g) cauliflower rice or 1 head cauliflower, riced (see note on page 108)
3 tablespoons (45 ml) coconut aminos
¼ teaspoon ground ginger
Bang Bang Sauce (page 33)

1. Heat 1 tablespoon (15 ml) of the sesame oil in a large nonstick skillet over medium-high heat.
2. Add the shrimp and cook until pink or opaque and the tails curl, flipping halfway through, about 3 minutes total. Remove the shrimp to a plate; set aside.
3. Crack the eggs into the skillet and scramble. Cook until fluffy, 2 to 3 minutes, and transfer to the plate with the shrimp.
4. Add the remaining 1½ teaspoons (7 ml) sesame oil to the hot skillet, along with green beans, carrots, shallot, scallion, and garlic. Cook, stirring, until the veggies are tender, 3 to 4 minutes.
5. Add the cauliflower rice and scrambled eggs back to the skillet and stir together until well combined and the cauliflower rice is cooked.
6. Return the shrimp to the skillet and add the coconut aminos and ginger, stirring to combine.
7. Divide the mixture among bowls and drizzle with the Bang Bang Sauce.

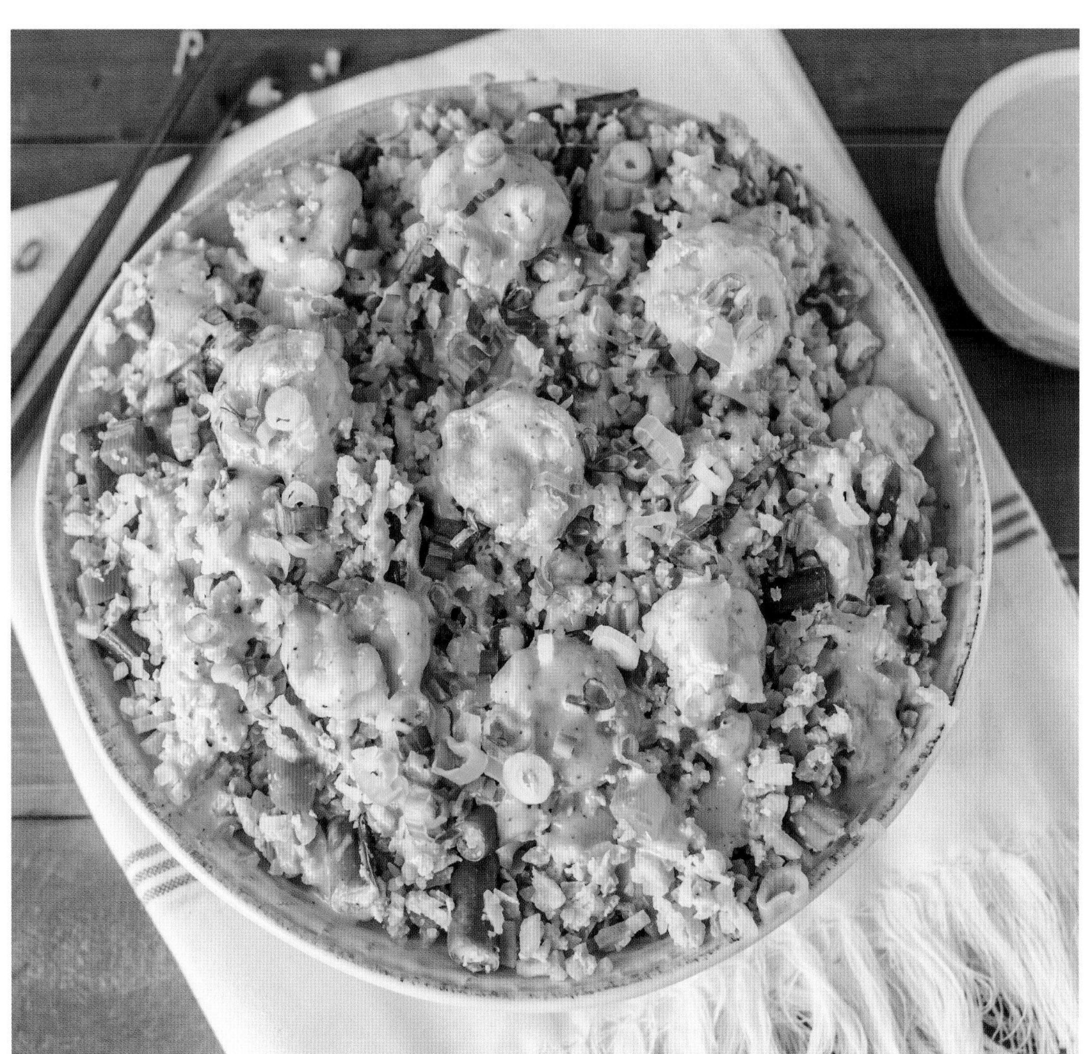

Basil Pesto Chicken Power Bowls

Power bowls are a great way to fuel your body in a healthy, yet satisfying, way. This chicken pesto bowl is such a simple recipe, but it will revolutionize your lunch or dinner.

SQUEAKY CLEAN PALEO / KETO PALEO / TRADITIONAL PALEO

Makes: 4 servings / **Prep Time:** 7 minutes / **Total Time:** 20 to 25 minutes

4 boneless, skinless chicken breasts (6 ounces [168 g] each)
4 vines with cherry tomatoes
1 tablespoon (15 ml) olive oil, plus more for drizzling
2 yellow squash, sliced
8 spears asparagus, trimmed
4 cups (560 g) cauliflower rice (see Note)
Sea salt and black pepper, to taste
½ cup (120 g) Basil Pesto (page 37)
Lemon slices, for garnish

1. Grease the grill and preheat to 400°F (200°C) or medium-high heat.
2. Place the chicken on the grill and cook until the internal temperature reaches 160°F (71°C), 5 to 8 minutes on each side, depending on the thickness of the breasts.
3. Place the tomatoes (on the vine) on a sheet of aluminum foil and drizzle with a little olive oil. Set it on the grill and cook until they become a little shriveled and soft, 5 to 6 minutes.
4. Right before the chicken is done, add the squash and asparagus to the grill and cook until tender and grill marks are visible, 2 to 3 minutes on each side. When ready, remove the asparagus to a cutting board and chop into 1-inch (2.5 cm) pieces.
5. Meanwhile, heat the olive oil in a large skillet over medium heat. Add the cauliflower rice, cover, and cook, stirring occasionally, until tender, 5 to 6 minutes. Sprinkle with a large pinch of salt and pepper.
6. Assemble the power bowls by adding 1 cup (140 g) cauliflower rice to each of 4 bowls. Add a chicken breast topped with 2 tablespoons (30 g) of the pesto. Set a vine of tomatoes, some squash, and asparagus pieces around the chicken. Serve with lemon slices.

RECIPE NOTES

If you are using a head of cauliflower, add the florets to a food processor and pulse until it becomes a rice-like consistency. Add the rice to a bowl along with ¼ cup (60 ml) water and microwave for 2 minutes. This will help make it tender and quicker to cook in step 5. You should have about 4 cups (560 g).

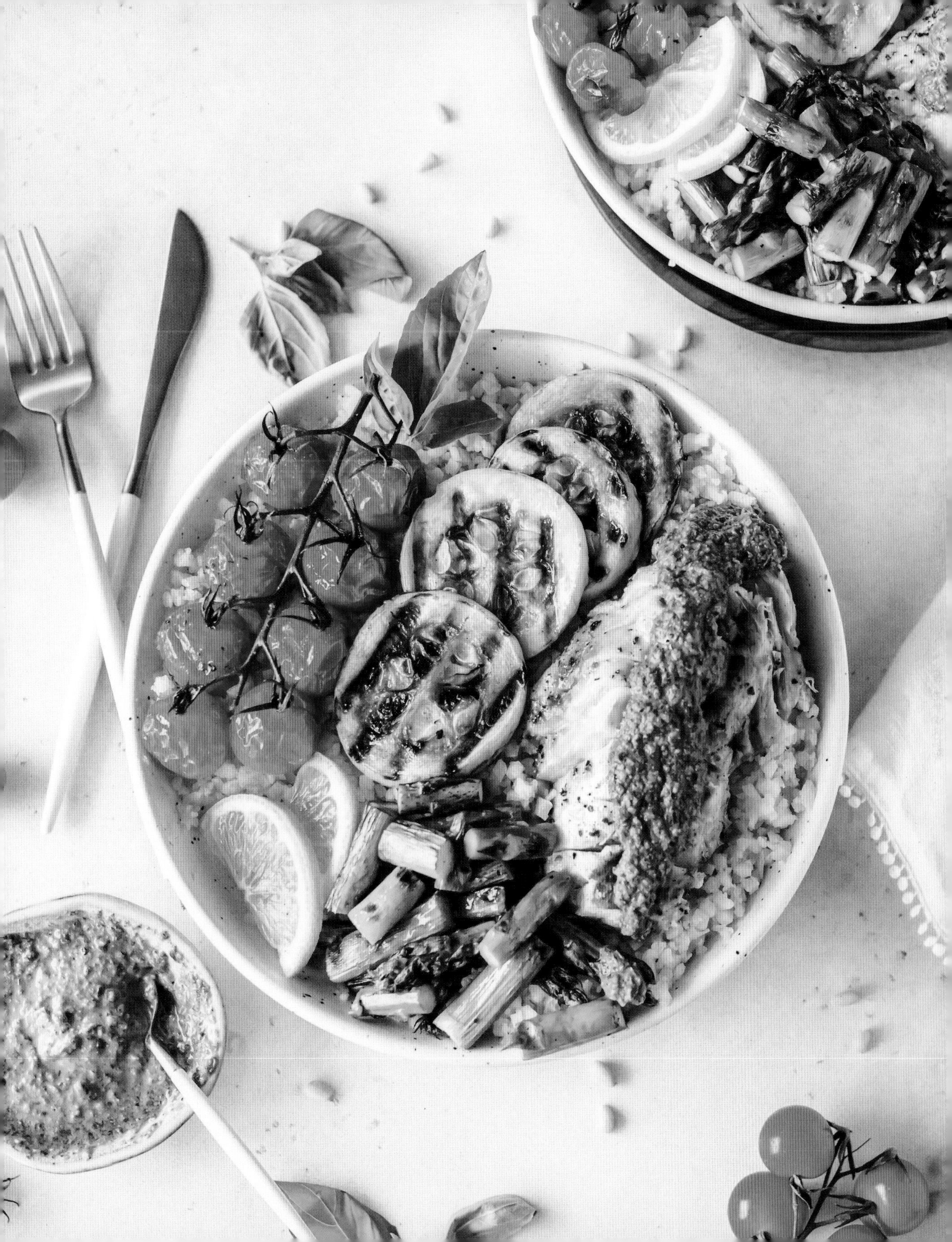

Sausage Skillet Stir-Fry

This recipe should be on a weekly rotation in your house because of how simple and delicious it is. It can be pulled together in 15 minutes or less and is extremely filling. Savory sausage, sautéed peppers, onions, cabbage, and cauliflower rice will keep you feeling full for hours. It's also great served with a dollop of Mac's Awesome Sauce (page 31) or Chili Lime Sauce (page 32).

SQUEAKY CLEAN PALEO / KETO PALEO / TRADITIONAL PALEO

Makes: 4 servings / **Prep Time:** 7 minutes / **Total Time:** 15 minutes

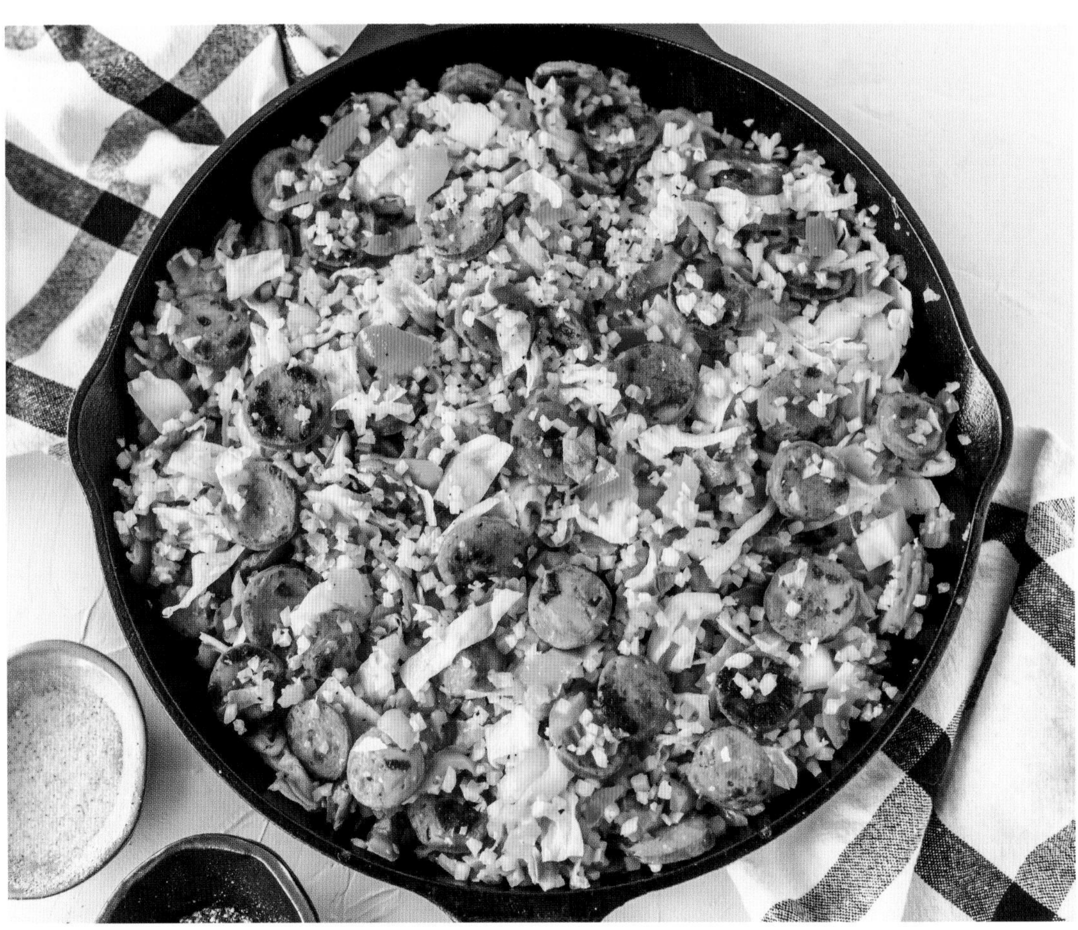

2 tablespoons (30 ml) olive oil, divided
1 clove garlic, minced
4 links chicken apple sausage, sliced ¼ inch (6 mm) thick
2 cups (180 g) chopped green cabbage
½ yellow onion, sliced
½ red bell pepper, sliced
½ green bell pepper, sliced
½ orange bell pepper, sliced
1 bag (12 ounces [336 g]) cauliflower rice or ½ head cauliflower, cut into florets (see Note)
3 tablespoons (45 ml) coconut aminos
Sea salt, to taste
¼ teaspoon black pepper
¼ teaspoon onion powder

---

1. Heat 1 tablespoon (15 ml) of the olive oil and the garlic in a large skillet over medium-high heat.
2. Add the sausage and cook, stirring occasionally, until cooked through, 3 to 4 minutes. Remove from the skillet to a plate.
3. Add the remaining 1 tablespoon (15 ml) olive oil to the skillet, along with the cabbage, onion, and bell peppers. Cook until tender, about 5 minutes.
4. Add the riced cauliflower, coconut aminos, salt, black pepper, and onion powder. Stir to combine and cook until the cauliflower is tender and hot, 2 to 3 minutes more.
5. Add the sausage back to the skillet and stir together.
6. Cook for another 2 minutes. Taste and add more salt, if needed.

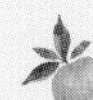

RECIPE NOTES

If you are using a head of cauliflower, add the florets to a food processor and pulse until it becomes a rice-like consistency. Add the rice to a bowl along with 2 tablespoons (30 ml) of water and microwave for 2 minutes. This will help make it tender and quicker to cook in step 4. You should have about 2 cups (280 g).

Philly Not-So-Cheesesteak Stuffed Peppers

These stuffed peppers are a spin on the traditional Philly cheesesteak sandwiches. They're filled with thinly sliced steak, mushrooms, and peppers and get a big dollop of Mac's Awesome Sauce. They're so good, you won't even miss the bread.

SQUEAKY CLEAN PALEO / KETO PALEO / TRADITIONAL PALEO

Makes: 8 to 10 servings / **Prep Time:** 10 minutes / **Total Time:** 35 minutes

- 4 or 5 green bell peppers, halved and seeded
- 2 tablespoons (30 ml) olive oil, divided
- 16 to 18 ounces (454 to 510 g) sirloin steak, thinly sliced against the grain
- 1 cup (70 g) sliced mushrooms
- 1 red bell pepper, seeded and thinly sliced
- 1 small red onion, thinly sliced
- ½ cup (120 ml) Mac's Awesome Sauce (page 37)
- Chopped fresh parsley, for garnish

1. Preheat the oven to 400°F (200°C or gas mark 6) and oil a rimmed baking sheet.
2. Place the halved green bell peppers cut-side up on the baking sheet. Bake until tender, about 20 minutes.
3. Meanwhile, heat 1 tablespoon (15 ml) of the olive oil in a large skillet over medium-high heat. Add the steak and cook until the desired doneness, 5 to 6 minutes. Remove the steak to a bowl; set aside.
4. Add the remaining 1 tablespoon (15 ml) olive oil to the hot skillet. Add the mushrooms, red bell pepper, and onion and cook until the veggies are tender, 4 to 5 minutes.
5. Add the steak slices back to the skillet and cook another minute or two to combine and warm through.
6. Remove the peppers from the oven and add a heaping spoonful of the veggie and meat mixture to each pepper. Once each pepper is filled, top each with 1 tablespoon (15 ml) of Mac's Awesome Sauce.
7. Return the peppers to the oven and bake until the sauce begins to bubble, another 2 to 3 minutes.
8. Sprinkle with the parsley before serving.

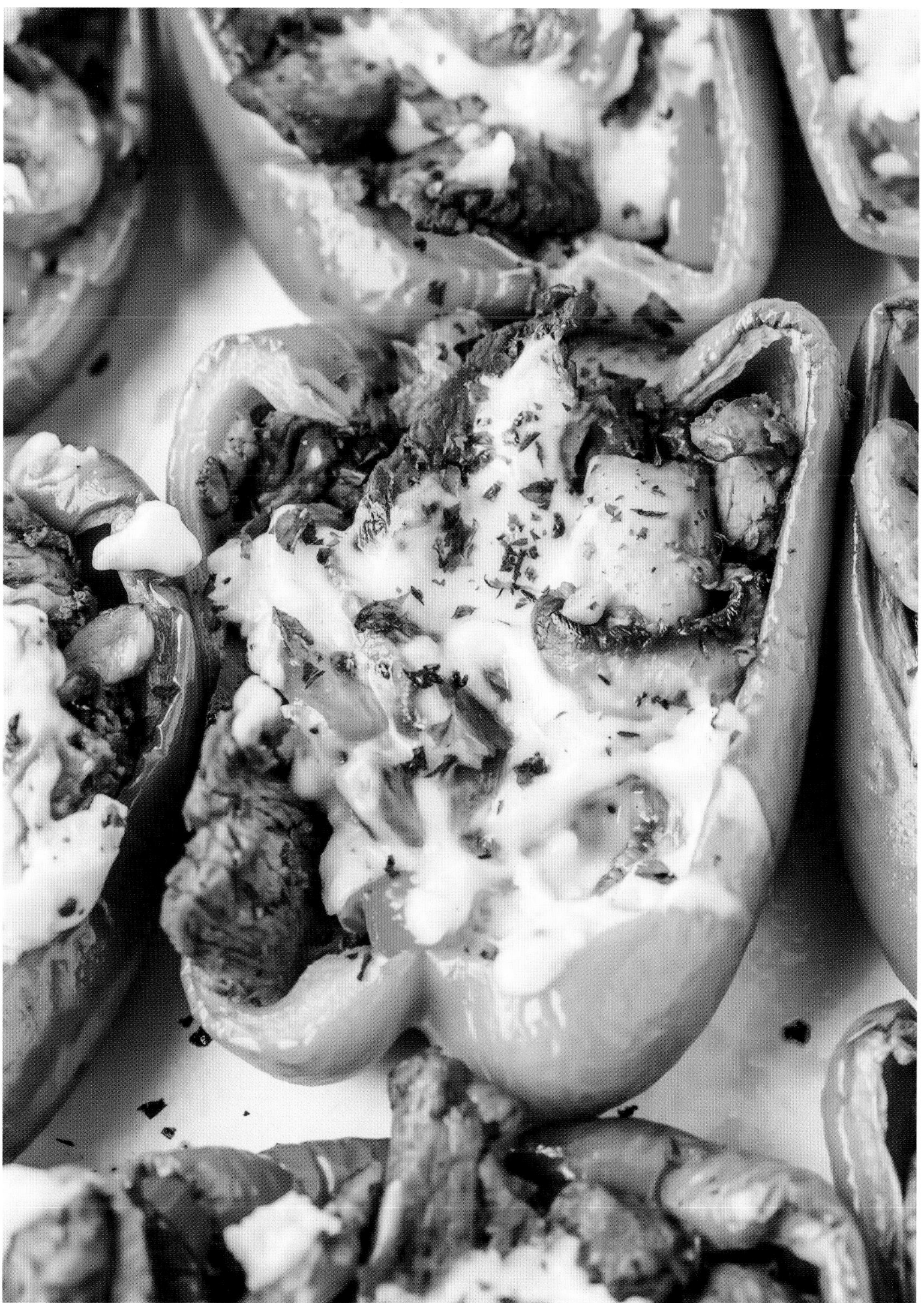

Tuscan Shrimp

This quick shrimp dish brings home the flavors of Tuscany: sun-dried tomatoes, spinach, and a delectable cream sauce. Serve with a beautiful side salad to make a complete meal.

SQUEAKY CLEAN PALEO / KETO PALEO / TRADITIONAL PALEO

Makes: 4 to 5 servings / **Prep Time:** 5 minutes / **Total Time:** 15 minutes

1 tablespoon (14 g) ghee
1½ pounds (680 g) jumbo peeled and deveined shrimp
1 cup (240 ml) compliant chicken broth
⅓ cup (80 ml) canned unsweetened coconut milk
1½ tablespoons (9 g) arrowroot powder or tapioca flour dissolved in 2 tablespoons (30 ml) water (see Note)
2 cups (60 g) baby spinach
¼ cup (27 g) no-sugar-added whole sun-dried tomatoes in olive oil
1 tablespoon (15 ml) lemon juice
Sea salt and black pepper to taste
Chopped fresh parsley, for garnish
1 bag (12 ounces [336 g]) cauliflower rice, steamed, or Cauliflower Mash (page 96) (optional)

1. Heat the ghee in a large skillet over medium heat until the ghee starts to sizzle. Add the shrimp and cook until pink or opaque and the tails curl, 3 to 4 minutes, flipping once. Remove the shrimp to a plate and set aside.
2. Add the broth and coconut milk to the skillet and stir together.
3. Add the arrowroot mixture and whisk until thickened, 2 to 3 minutes.
4. Add the spinach, tomatoes, and lemon juice. Stir together and add salt and pepper to taste.
5. Return the shrimp to the skillet and simmer over low heat for 2 minutes to combine and warm through.
6. Sprinkle with the parsley and serve over cauliflower rice or mash, if desired.

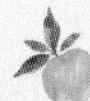

RECIPE NOTES

The gravy won't be as thick as when made with regular flour. It is the consistency of a thicker soup. Feel free to add less broth to make it thicker, or experiment with adding a little more tapioca flour. Remember that it will begin to thicken as it heats. To make this Keto Paleo, replace the tapioca flour with 1½ tablespoons (14 g) gelatin or ¼ teaspoon xanthan gum.

Hibachi Chicken Skewers and Veggies

Bring the hibachi grill to your kitchen with these chicken skewers served over grilled veggies. Drizzled with Bang Bang Sauce, they taste identical to what you'd find at a restaurant.

SQUEAKY CLEAN PALEO / KETO PALEO / TRADITIONAL PALEO

Makes: 4 servings / **Prep Time:** 10 minutes / **Total Time:** 20 to 25 minutes

---

CHICKEN SKEWERS

12 chicken breast tenderloins
Sea salt and black pepper
Four 10- or 12-inch (25 or 30 cm) wooden skewers
1 tablespoon (15 ml) olive oil
4 tablespoons (60 ml) coconut aminos

HIBACHI VEGGIES

1 tablespoon (15 ml) olive oil
3 small zucchini, halved lengthwise, then sliced
3 carrots, sliced
1 cup (70 g) sliced mushrooms
1 small yellow onion, cut into thick chunks
3 tablespoons (45 ml) coconut aminos
½ teaspoon ground ginger
Sea salt and black pepper to taste

Bang Bang Sauce (page 33)

CHICKEN SKEWERS

1. Sprinkle the chicken tenders with salt and pepper and thread 3 tenders onto each skewer.
2. Heat the olive oil in a large skillet or grill pan over medium-high heat. Add the chicken skewers.
3. Pour 1 tablespoon (15 ml) of the coconut aminos over each skewer. Cook until the chicken is golden and the juices run clear, about 6 minutes on each side.

HIBACHI VEGGIES

1. Heat the olive oil in a large skillet over medium-high heat. Add the zucchini, carrots, mushrooms, onion, coconut aminos, ginger, and a pinch of salt and pepper. Cook, stirring occasionally, until tender, 6 minutes.
2. Divide the veggies among 4 plates and top each with a chicken skewer. Drizzle with the Bang Bang Sauce.

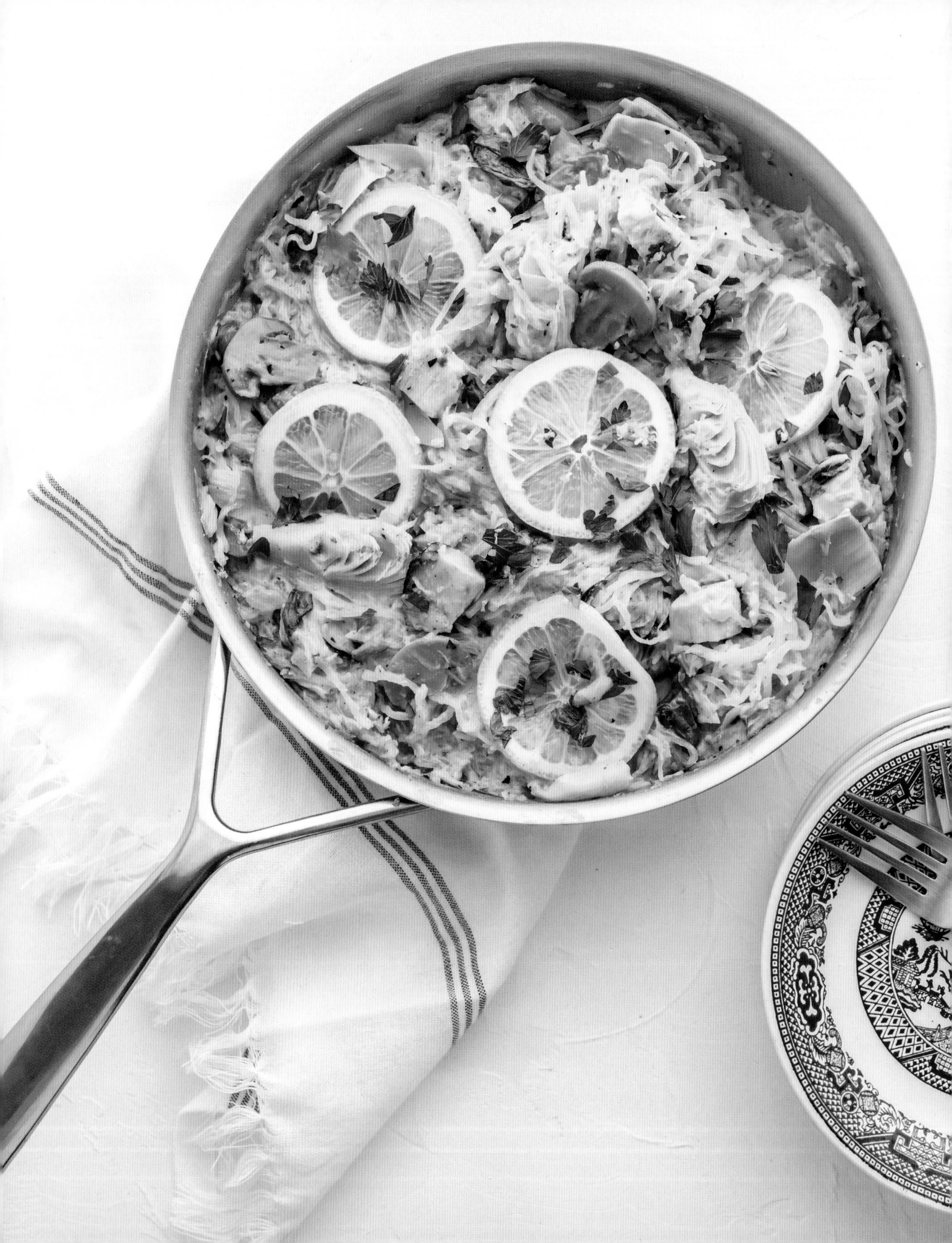

Spinach-Artichoke Chicken Skillet

One-skillet dishes save lives because cleanup is a breeze. This skillet dinner can be ready in 30 minutes or less by using an electric pressure cooker to cook the spaghetti squash.

SQUEAKY CLEAN PALEO / KETO PALEO / TRADITIONAL PALEO

Makes: 4 servings / **Prep Time:** 10 minutes / **Total Time:** 15 minutes + time to cook the squash

---

1 small (3- to 4-pound [1.3 to 1.8 kg]) spaghetti squash
Olive oil, for the squash
1 tablespoon (14 g) ghee
1 pound (454 g) boneless, skinless chicken breasts
1 can (4 ounces [112 g]) sliced mushrooms, drained
1 cup (30 g) baby spinach
4 artichoke hearts, quartered
1 clove garlic, minced
1 cup (240 ml) compliant chicken broth
½ cup (120 ml) canned unsweetened coconut milk
1 lemon, ½ juiced, ½ sliced for garnish
1½ tablespoons (9 g) tapioca flour
½ teaspoon sea salt
¼ teaspoon black pepper
¼ teaspoon onion powder
Chopped fresh parsley, for garnish

COOKING SPAGHETTI SQUASH IN THE OVEN

Heat the oven to 400°F (200°C or gas mark 6). Slice the squash in half lengthwise and scoop out the seeds. Drizzle the halves with olive oil and sprinkle with sea salt. Place cut-side down on a baking sheet and roast until tender, 45 to 50 minutes. Let cool slightly, then use a fork to shred the squash flesh.

COOKING SPAGHETTI SQUASH IN THE ELECTRIC PRESSURE COOKER

Pierce the squash all over with a paring knife. Place a trivet or steamer basket in the bottom of the electric pressure cooker, set the squash on top, and add 1 cup (240 ml) water to the bottom. Cook on high pressure for 15 minutes. Use instant release to release the cooker's pressure. Remove the squash and let cool slightly. Halve lengthwise, drizzle with olive oil, and sprinkle with salt. Shred the squash flesh with a fork.

SPINACH-ARTICHOKE CHICKEN

1. Prepare the spaghetti squash.
2. Heat the ghee in a large skillet over medium-high heat until it sizzles.
3. Add the chicken and cook until the internal temperature reaches 160°F (71°C), about 5 minutes on each side. Remove the chicken to a cutting board, let cool slightly, and then chop.
4. To the hot skillet, add the mushrooms, spinach, artichoke hearts, and garlic. Cook until heated through and the spinach wilts, 2 to 3 minutes. Add the chicken back to the skillet, stirring to combine.
5. Stir in the spaghetti squash and mix together.
6. In a medium bowl, whisk together the broth, coconut milk, lemon juice, tapioca flour, salt, black pepper, and onion powder.
7. Pour the broth mixture into the skillet and stir to combine well.
8. Reduce the heat to low and simmer until the sauce begins to thicken, about 3 minutes.
9. Garnish with the parsley and lemon slices before serving. For a cheesy texture and taste, sprinkle the top of this skillet with a few shakes of nutritional yeast.

Hawaiian BBQ Chicken Wraps with Ranch Coleslaw

Chicken can get so boring sometimes. That's when these Hawaiian wraps topped with grilled pineapple and ranch-drenched coleslaw swoop in to save the day.

SQUEAKY CLEAN PALEO / TRADITIONAL PALEO

Makes: 4 servings / **Prep Time:** 10 minutes / **Total Time:** 30 to 35 minutes

- 1 tablespoon (15 ml) avocado or olive oil
- 4 medium boneless, skinless chicken breasts (6 ounces [168 g] each)
- 4 slices pineapple
- 3 cups (210 g) packaged coleslaw mix
- ¼ cup (60 ml) Ranch Dressing (page 30)
- Splash of rice vinegar
- 4 tablespoons (60 ml) BBQ Sauce (page 35) or compliant BBQ sauce, divided
- 8 butter lettuce leaves
- 4 large red onion slices

1. Preheat the oven to 425°F (220°C or gas mark 7).
2. Heat the oil in a large oven-safe skillet over medium-high heat. Add the chicken and cook for 4 minutes on each side.
3. Transfer the skillet to the oven and cook until the internal temperature reaches 160°F (71°C), about 10 minutes.
4. Meanwhile, heat a grill or another skillet over medium-high heat. Add the pineapple and cook until tender or until the desired doneness. Set aside.
5. In a medium bowl, combine the coleslaw mix, dressing, and splash of rice vinegar, mixing with a spoon until well combined.
6. Remove the chicken from the oven and, using a basting brush, coat each chicken breast with the BBQ sauce, 1 tablespoon (15 ml) each.
7. Assemble the wraps by starting with a lettuce cup on the bottom and building with a chicken breast, ¾ cup (25 g) ranch coleslaw, 1 pineapple ring, and 1 red onion slice. Top everything with another lettuce cup.

RECIPE NOTES

You can also wrap each chicken wrap in parchment paper to hold everything together

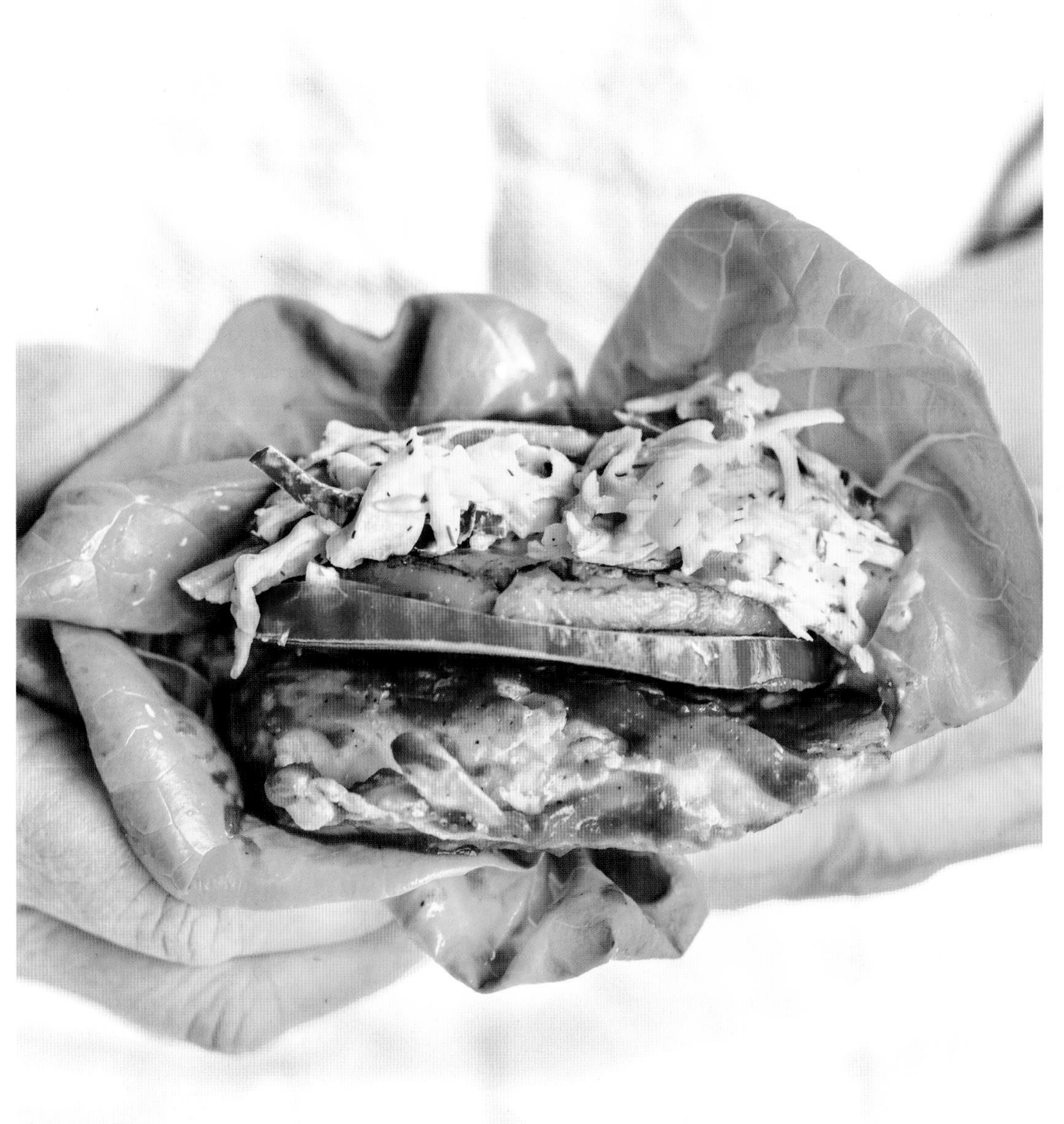

Stuffed Mexican Spaghetti Squash

This Mexican-style spaghetti squash is filled with all the flavors you'd expect, such as fire-roasted tomatoes, shredded pork, jalapeños, onions, and lime juice. It's even more perfect when served with sliced avocados and fresh salsa.

SQUEAKY CLEAN PALEO / TRADITIONAL PALEO

Makes: 4 servings / **Prep Time:** 10 minutes / **Total Time:** 30 minutes + time to cook the squash

1 large spaghetti squash (5 to 6 pounds [2.3 to 2.7 kg])
Olive oil, for the squash
3 cups (420 g) cooked Shredded Pork (page 140)
1 can (14.5 ounces [406 g]) fire-roasted diced tomatoes, drained
⅓ cup (55 g) chopped onion
¼ cup (60 ml) canned unsweetened coconut milk
2½ tablespoons (15 g) almond flour
2½ tablespoons (15 g) taco seasoning (recipe follows)
2 tablespoons (8 g) nutritional yeast
2 tablespoons (18 g) chopped jalapeños
1 tablespoon (15 ml) lime juice
For garnish: 1 large sliced avocado, compliant salsa, jalapeño slices, and chopped cilantro

TACO SEASONING

1½ tablespoons (9 g) chili powder
2 teaspoons ground cumin
1 teaspoon sea salt
1 teaspoon black pepper
½ teaspoon dried oregano
½ teaspoon onion powder
½ teaspoon garlic powder
¼ teaspoon paprika

COOKING SPAGHETTI SQUASH IN THE OVEN

Heat the oven to 400°F (200°C or gas mark 6). Slice the squash in half lengthwise and scoop out the seeds. Drizzle the halves with olive oil and sprinkle with sea salt. Place cut-side down on a baking sheet and roast until tender, 55 to 60 minutes. Let cool slightly, then use a fork to shred the squash flesh.

COOKING SPAGHETTI SQUASH IN THE ELECTRIC PRESSURE COOKER

Pierce the squash all over with a paring knife. Place a trivet or steamer basket in the bottom of the electric pressure cooker, set the squash on top, and add 1 cup (240 ml) water to the bottom. (If the squash is too large to fit, cut it in half.) Cook on high pressure for 15 minutes. Use instant release to release the cooker's pressure. Remove the squash and let cool slightly. Halve lengthwise, drizzle with olive oil, and sprinkle with salt. Shred the squash flesh with a fork.

TACO SEASONING

To a small jar, add the chili powder, cumin, salt, pepper, oregano, onion powder, garlic powder, and paprika. Cap the jar and shake until well combined. (Store any extra to sprinkle on eggs or guacamole.)

STUFFED SQUASH

1. Prepare the squash, reserving the shells once the flesh is shredded.
2. Preheat the oven to 350°F (180°C or gas mark 4).
3. Transfer the cooked strands of squash to a large mixing bowl, along with the pork, tomatoes, onion, coconut milk, almond flour, taco seasoning, nutritional yeast, jalapeños, and lime juice. Mix together until well combined.
4. Place the 2 shells of the spaghetti squash on a baking sheet and transfer the squash mixture back into the shells.
5. Bake until heated through and bubbling, 15 to 20 minutes.
6. Garnish with the avocado, salsa, jalapeño, and cilantro.

RECIPE NOTES

This is a great recipe to make if you have leftover shredded pork from a previous dinner. If not, luckily the pork is a snap to make in the slow cooker if you set it before you leave for work in the morning, or the electric pressure cooker, if you need to make it when you come home. You can also find premade compliant shredded pork at some grocery stores.

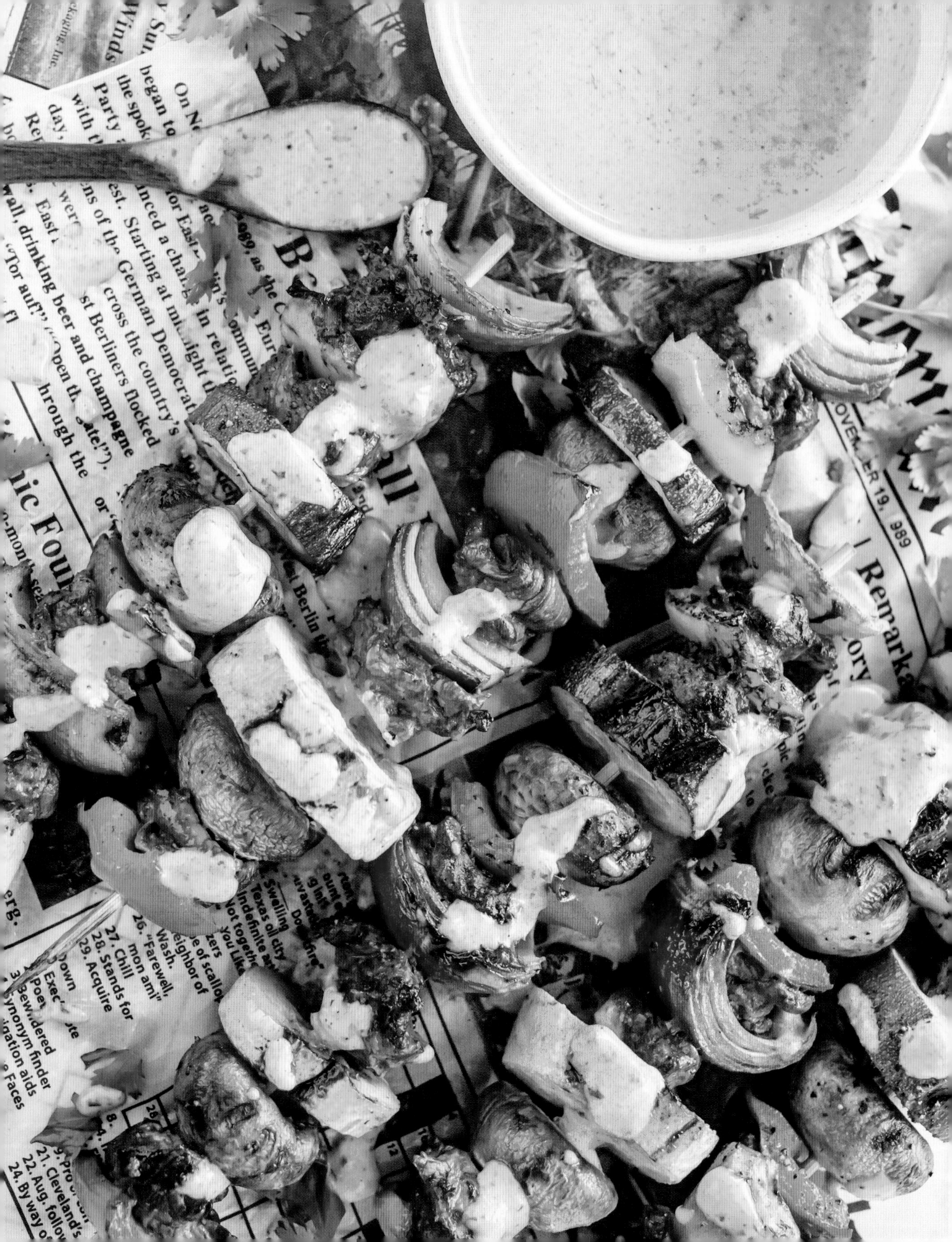

Steak Kabobs with Southwest Sauce

Steak kabobs scream "summer," but this recipe is good year-round. Layered with juicy sirloin steak bites and tender veggies, they're drenched in a smoky, slightly spicy sauce that will steal the show.

SQUEAKY CLEAN PALEO / KETO PALEO / TRADITIONAL PALEO

Makes: 4 to 5 servings / **Prep Time:** 10 minutes / **Total Time:** 30 minutes + marinating time

- ⅓ cup (80 ml) olive oil
- ¼ cup (60 ml) coconut aminos
- Juice of 1 lemon
- 2 cloves garlic, minced
- 2 teaspoons dried parsley
- 1½ pounds (680 g) sirloin steak, cut into 1-inch (2.5 cm) cubes
- Four or five 10-inch (25 cm) wooden skewers
- 1 medium zucchini, cut into 1-inch (2.5 cm) chunks
- 1 medium yellow squash, cut into 1-inch (2.5 cm) chunks
- 1 red bell pepper, cut into 1-inch (2.5 cm) pieces
- 1 red onion, cut into 1-inch (2.5 cm) cubes (about 3 onion layers each)
- 1 cup (70 g) whole mushrooms
- Southwest Sauce (page 34)

1. In a medium bowl, whisk together the olive oil, coconut aminos, lemon juice, garlic, and parsley. Transfer to a 1-gallon (3.6 L) resealable plastic bag.
2. Add the steak, seal, and gently toss to coat the steak. Set aside to marinate for 30 minutes or up to 1 hour.
3. Preheat the grill to medium-high.
4. Thread the steak cubes onto the skewers, alternating with pieces of zucchini, squash, bell pepper, onion, and mushrooms. (Discard the marinade.) Transfer the kabobs to the grill.
5. Cook, turning the kabobs often, until the meat is well browned and the vegetables are tender, about 15 minutes.
6. Divide the kabobs among plates and drizzle each with Southwest Sauce before serving.

RECIPE NOTES

To prevent the skewers from burning, soak them in water while the steak marinates.

Hamburger Steaks

Nothing says "family dinner" like skillet hamburger steaks. These juicy burger patties bathe in a broth that is packed with garlic, sautéed onions, and mushrooms. For a complete meal, serve with Cauliflower Mash (page 96) or Smashed Sweet Potato Slices (page 92).

SQUEAKY CLEAN PALEO / KETO PALEO / TRADITIONAL PALEO

Makes: 6 servings / **Prep Time:** 10 minutes / **Total Time:** 25 minutes

- 2 pounds (910 g) 90/10 ground beef
- ¾ teaspoon sea salt, divided
- ½ teaspoon black pepper, divided
- 1 tablespoon (15 ml) olive oil
- 1 teaspoon ghee
- 1 small onion, sliced
- 1 can (8 ounces [224 g]) sliced mushrooms, drained
- 2 cups (480 ml) compliant beef broth
- ¼ teaspoon onion powder
- ¼ teaspoon garlic powder
- 1 teaspoon coarsely chopped fresh parsley

1. Gently form the ground beef into 6 hamburger patties. Indent the middle of each patty with your thumb to help keep the form while cooking. Sprinkle the patties on both sides with ½ teaspoon of the salt and ¼ teaspoon of the pepper.
2. Heat the olive oil in a large skillet over medium-high heat. Add the patties, leaving space between them.
3. Cook the patties until the desired doneness, or when the internal temperature reaches 160°F (71°C), 5 to 6 minutes per side. Remove the burgers to a plate.
4. Add the ghee to the skillet, along with the sliced onion and mushrooms. Stir together and cook until the onion softens, 3 to 4 minutes.
5. Add the broth, onion powder, garlic powder, remaining ¼ teaspoon salt, and remaining ¼ teaspoon pepper. Cook until heated through, 1 to 2 minutes.
6. Return the hamburger patties to the skillet and use a spoon to cover them with the sauce and veggies.
7. Sprinkle with the parsley before serving.

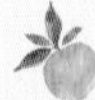

RECIPE NOTES

I did not use a thickening agent with this dish because the broth is so good without it. If you want the broth to be thick, add 1½ tablespoons (9 g) tapioca flour dissolved in 2 tablespoons (30 ml) water to the broth mixture in step 5. To make this Keto, use ¼ teaspoon xanthan gum or 1½ tablespoons (14 g) of gelatin to thicken.

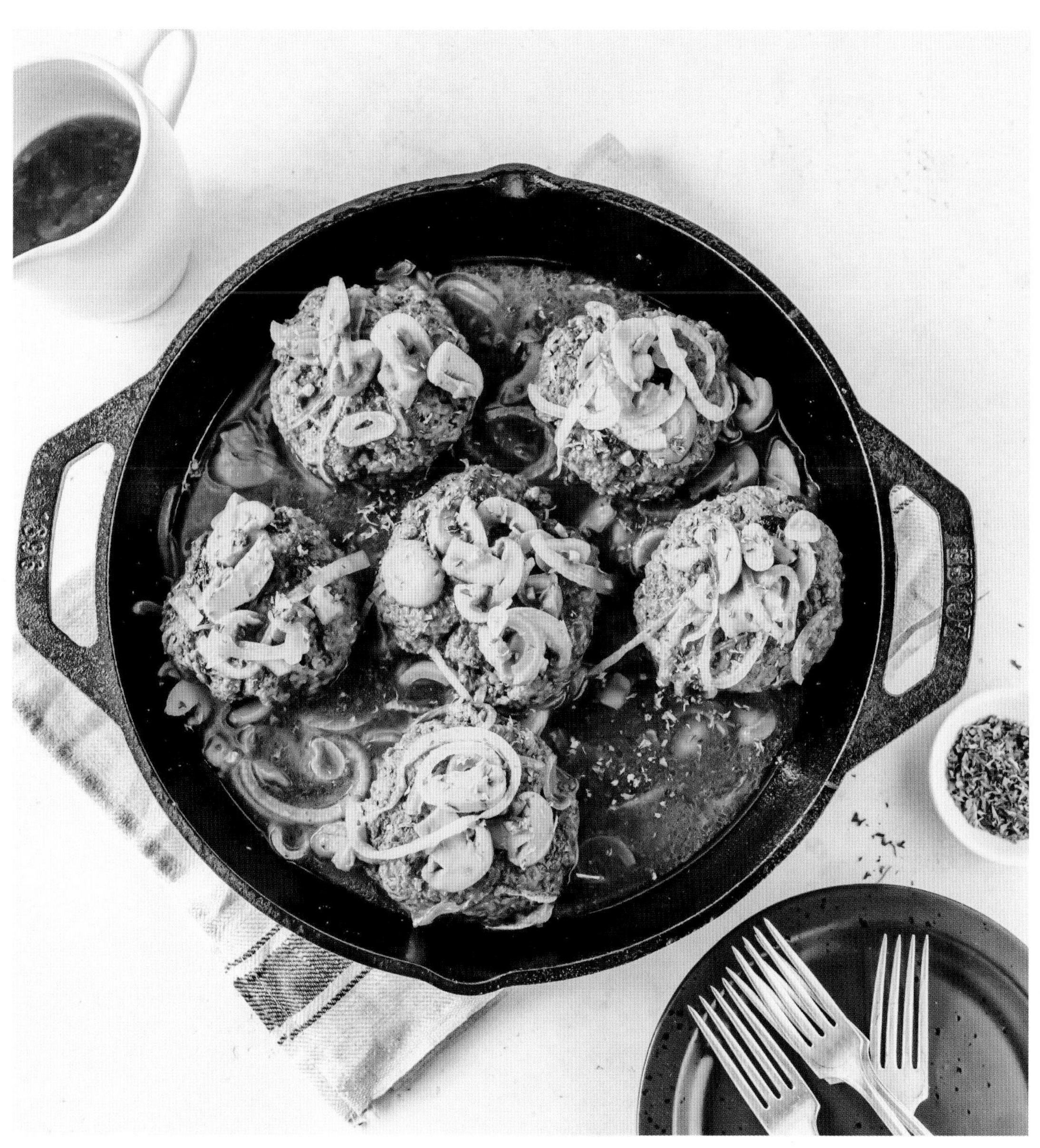

Tuna Cakes with Lemon-Dill Aioli

Incorporating tuna into family meals can really help on a budget. These tuna patties are drizzled with a lemon aioli. Use for an easy dinner or make a big batch on Sunday and use for meals throughout the week.

SQUEAKY CLEAN PALEO / KETO PALEO / TRADITIONAL PALEO

Makes: 8 to 10 patties / **Prep Time:** 8 minutes / **Total Time:** 20 minutes

TUNA PATTIES

5 cans (5 ounces [140 g]) tuna packed in water, drained
1 cup (96 g) almond flour
1 large egg
¼ cup (40 g) diced yellow onion
3 tablespoons (18 g) chopped scallion
1 tablespoon (15 ml) lemon juice
1 tablespoon (2 g) dried chives
1 tablespoon (2 g) dried parsley
2 teaspoons Dijon mustard
2 teaspoons compliant hot sauce
1 teaspoon lemon zest
½ teaspoon garlic powder
Sea salt and black pepper
1½ tablespoons (23 ml) olive oil
1 tablespoon (14 g) ghee
Lemon wedges, for serving (optional)

LEMON-DILL AIOLI

1 cup (240 g) Mayo (page 28) or compliant mayonnaise
Juice of 1 lemon
2 teaspoons dried dill weed
2 cloves garlic
1½ teaspoons lemon zest
1 teaspoon dried chives
Sea salt, to taste
¼ teaspoon black pepper

TUNA PATTIES

1. In a large mixing bowl, combine the tuna, almond flour, egg, onion, scallion, lemon juice, chives, parsley, mustard, hot sauce, lemon zest, garlic powder, and a pinch of salt and pepper. Mix together until well combined.
2. Form the tuna mixture into 1½-inch (3.8 cm)-thick patties (or desired size).
3. Heat the olive oil and ghee in a large cast-iron or nonstick skillet over medium-high heat. Gently add the patties and cook until browned, 4 minutes on each side.
4. Serve with a dollop of the Lemon-Dill Aioli and a squeeze of lemon over the top, if desired.

LEMON-DILL AIOLI

Add the mayo, lemon juice, dill, garlic, lemon zest, chives, salt, and pepper to a wide-mouth mason jar. Use an immersion blender to mix together until thick and creamy. (You may also make this in a regular blender.)

Creamy Mushroom and Bacon Chicken Thighs

These perfect one-skillet chicken thighs are drenched in a creamy mushroom-garlic sauce and topped with crisp bacon. This meal can be ready in 15 minutes or less and is great served over Cauliflower Mash (page 96).

SQUEAKY CLEAN PALEO / KETO PALEO / TRADITIONAL PALEO

Makes: 4 to 5 servings / **Prep Time:** 5 minutes / **Total Time:** 15 minutes

- 1 tablespoon (15 ml) olive oil
- 4 or 5 large bone-in, skin-on chicken thighs
- 1 teaspoon sea salt
- ½ teaspoon black pepper
- ½ teaspoon garlic powder
- 1 tablespoon (14 g) ghee
- 2 cans (4 ounces [112 g]) mushrooms, drained
- ½ large sweet onion, thinly sliced
- 2 cloves garlic, minced
- 1½ cups (360 ml) compliant chicken broth
- 2 tablespoons (30 ml) canned unsweetened coconut milk
- ½ teaspoon onion powder
- ¼ teaspoon sea salt (more to taste)
- ¼ teaspoon black pepper
- 1½ tablespoons (9 g) tapioca flour dissolved in 2 tablespoons (30 ml) water
- 2 pieces cooked compliant bacon, chopped
- 3 tablespoons (12 g) chopped fresh parsley

1. Heat the olive oil in a large skillet over medium-high heat.
2. Pat each chicken thigh dry with a paper towel, then coat each thigh with a mixture of the salt, pepper, and garlic powder.
3. Add the chicken to the skillet and cook until the juices run clear and the internal temperature is 160°F (71°C), 7 to 8 minutes on each side.
4. Remove the chicken to a plate but keep the drippings in the skillet.
5. Add the ghee and when it sizzles, add the mushrooms, onion, and garlic.
6. Cook until the onion browns, 2 to 3 minutes. Then add the broth, coconut milk, onion powder, salt, and pepper. Stir until heated through.
7. Turn the heat to low. Add the tapioca mixture and whisk until thickened. (It will begin to thicken as it heats up; it won't happen instantly.)
8. Once thick, add the chicken thighs back to the gravy and cook for another 3 to 4 minutes.
9. Serve topped with crispy bacon and fresh parsley for garnish.

RECIPE NOTES

For Keto, use ¼ teaspoon xanthan gum or 1½ tablespoons (14 g) of gelatin to thicken.

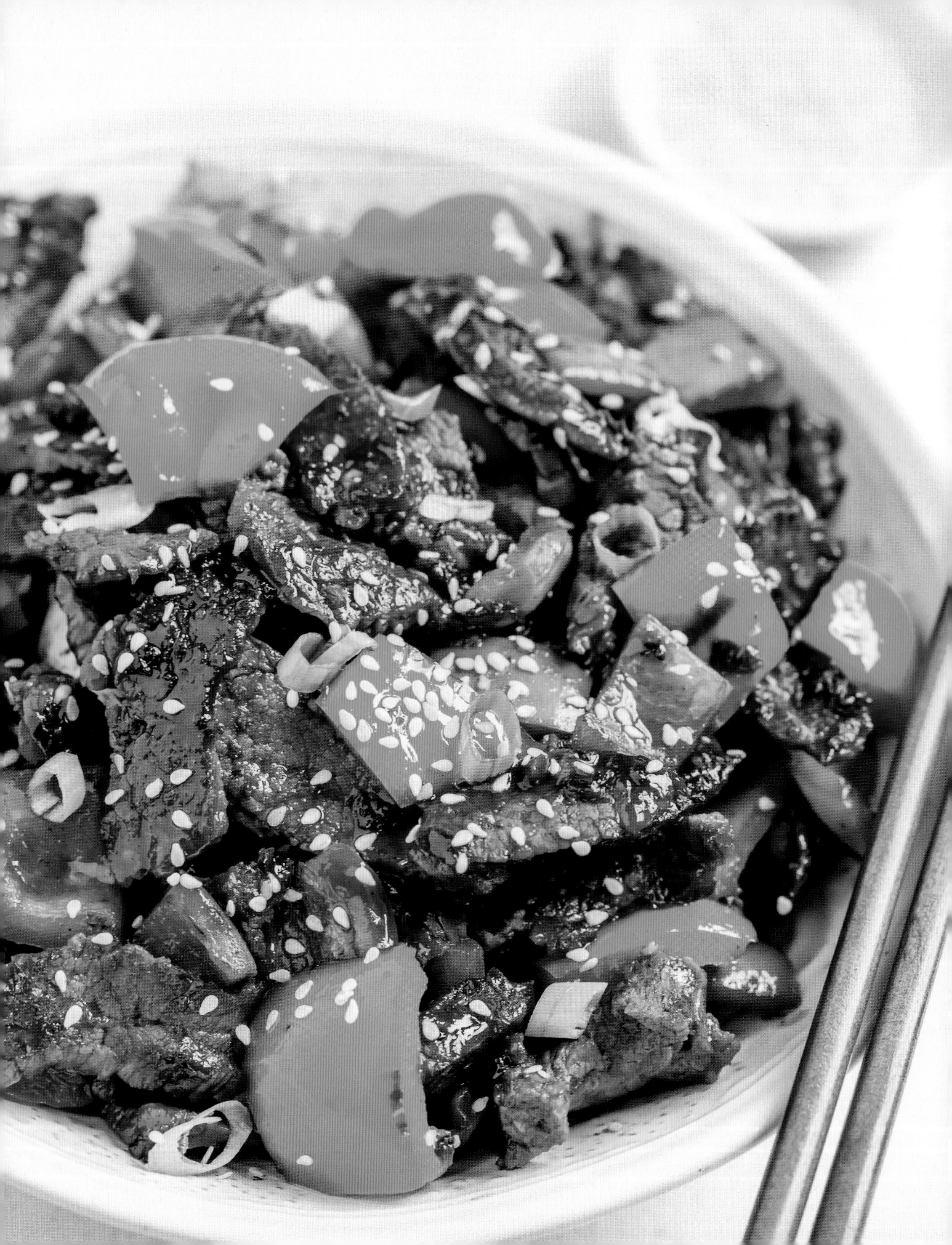

Quick Pepper Steak Stir-Fry

This Asian-inspired Paleo pepper steak stir-fry is perfect for when you're craving Chinese takeout—and it's about as quick to make as it would be to order. Serve it over cauliflower rice to make this a complete takeout copycat meal.

SQUEAKY CLEAN PALEO / KETO PALEO / TRADITIONAL PALEO

Makes: 4 servings / **Prep Time:** 5 minutes / **Total Time:** 15 minutes

---

1 tablespoon (15 ml) olive oil
1 red bell pepper, cut into 1-inch (2.5 cm) squares
1 green bell pepper, cut into 1-inch (2.5 cm) squares
1½ pounds (680 g) flank steak, thinly sliced against the grain into ½ by 4-inch (1.3 by 10 cm) strips
Sea salt and black pepper
2 cloves garlic, minced
½ cup (120 ml) coconut aminos
1½ tablespoons (23 ml) rice wine vinegar
1 tablespoon (15 ml) sesame oil
1 teaspoon tapioca flour
½ teaspoon ground ginger
¼ teaspoon onion powder
¼ teaspoon black pepper
Sliced scallions, for garnish
Sesame seeds, for garnish

---

1. Heat the olive oil in a large skillet over medium-high heat.
2. Add the bell peppers and cook until tender, 3 to 4 minutes. Remove to a dish and set aside.
3. Sprinkle the steak with salt and pepper. Add to the skillet, along with the garlic. Cook, stirring frequently, until the steak is tender, about 6 minutes.
4. Meanwhile, in a small bowl, whisk together the coconut aminos, rice wine vinegar, sesame oil, tapioca, ginger, onion powder, and black pepper.
5. Add the sauce and the bell peppers to the skillet. Simmer until the sauce thickens, 3 minutes.
6. Divide among bowls and garnish with scallions and sesame seeds.

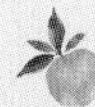

RECIPE NOTES

To make this Keto, replace the tapioca with 1½ tablespoons (14 g) gelatin or ¼ teaspoon xanthan gum to thicken.

Teriyaki Salmon

This baked salmon is tender and flavorful and takes only 15 minutes to make. It can serve as the perfect healthy weeknight meal.

SQUEAKY CLEAN PALEO / KETO PALEO / TRADITIONAL PALEO

Makes: 4 servings / **Prep Time:** 5 minutes / **Total Time:** 15 minutes

---

TERIYAKI SAUCE

¾ cup (180 ml) coconut aminos
¼ cup (60 ml) fresh squeezed orange juice
2 tablespoons (30 ml) pineapple juice
2 tablespoons (30 ml) sesame oil
1 clove garlic, minced
¼ teaspoon ground ginger
1 tablespoon (6 g) tapioca flour dissolved in 1½ tablespoons (23 ml) water

SALMON

4 salmon fillets (4 ounces [112 g] each)
1 tablespoon (15 ml) olive oil
2 tablespoons (30 g) coarse sea salt
1 bunch asparagus, trimmed
Chopped scallions, for garnish
Sesame seeds, for garnish
Microgreens, for garnish
4 cups (560 g) cauliflower rice, cooked

TERIYAKI SAUCE

1. In a small saucepan over medium heat, whisk together the coconut aminos, orange juice, pineapple juice, sesame oil, garlic, and ginger.
2. Once the mixture comes to a slow boil, add the tapioca mixture and whisk to combine.
3. Turn the heat to low. As it continues to heat, the sauce will become thicker.
4. Once thick, remove from the heat.

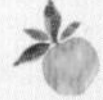

RECIPE NOTES

For Keto, replace the tapioca with 1½ tablespoons (14 g) gelatin or ¼ teaspoon xanthan gum to thicken.

SALMON

1. Preheat the oven to 350°F (180°C or gas mark 4) and line a baking sheet with aluminum foil.
2. Place the salmon on the baking sheet and drizzle the olive oil on each fillet.
3. Bake until the salmon is sizzling, 10 minutes.
4. Meanwhile, bring 8 cups (2 L) water and the salt to a boil in a large saucepan. Prepare a large bowl with ice and water. Add the asparagus to the saucepan and boil until crisp-tender, 3 minutes. Remove the asparagus to the ice water and let cool for 1 minute.
5. Remove the salmon from the oven and brush the teriyaki sauce on each fillet.
6. Garnish with the scallions, sesame seeds, and microgreens.
7. Serve with the asparagus and cauliflower rice.

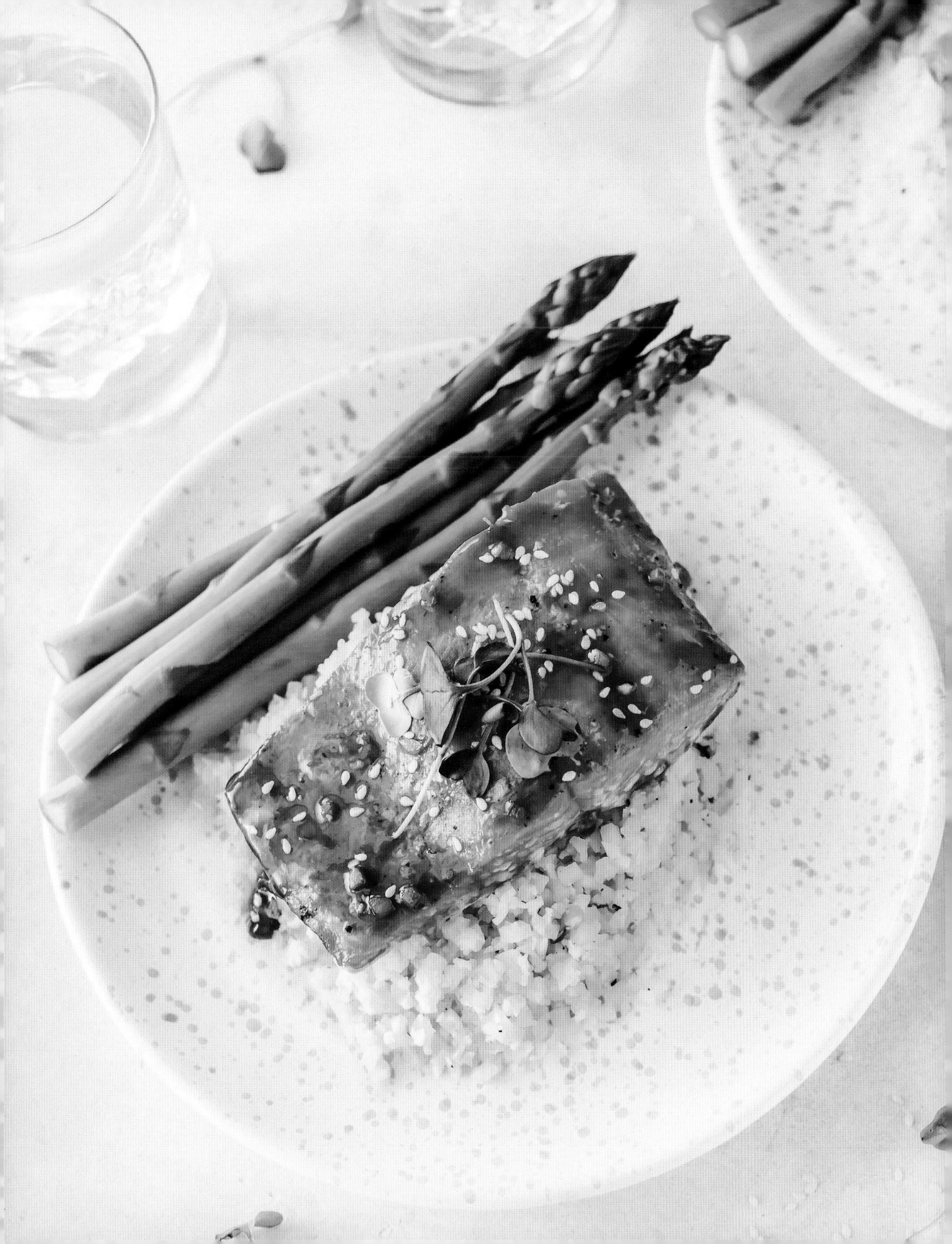

Cilantro-Lime Butterfly Chicken with Sweet Potato Fries

Roasting a whole chicken is a great way to save time in the kitchen, and a vibrant cilantro-lime marinade totally transforms this dish. Serve it with sweet potato fries made in the air fryer for a complete meal that's ready in about an hour.

SQUEAKY CLEAN PALEO / KETO PALEO / TRADITIONAL PALEO

Makes: 4 servings / **Prep Time:** 15 minutes / **Total Time:** 1 hour 15 minutes + rest time

---

MARINADE AND CHICKEN

2 handfuls fresh cilantro (about 2 cups [32 g]), plus more for garnish
⅓ cup (80 ml) light olive oil
Juice of 1 lime
2 cloves garlic
1 teaspoon sea salt
½ teaspoon black pepper
¼ teaspoon onion powder
1 whole chicken (5 pounds [2.3 kg])
1 lime, cut into wedges

SWEET POTATO FRIES

2 large sweet potatoes, cut into ¼-inch (6 mm)-thick fries
1½ tablespoons (23 ml) olive oil
1 teaspoon sea salt
½ teaspoon garlic powder
½ teaspoon cracked black pepper

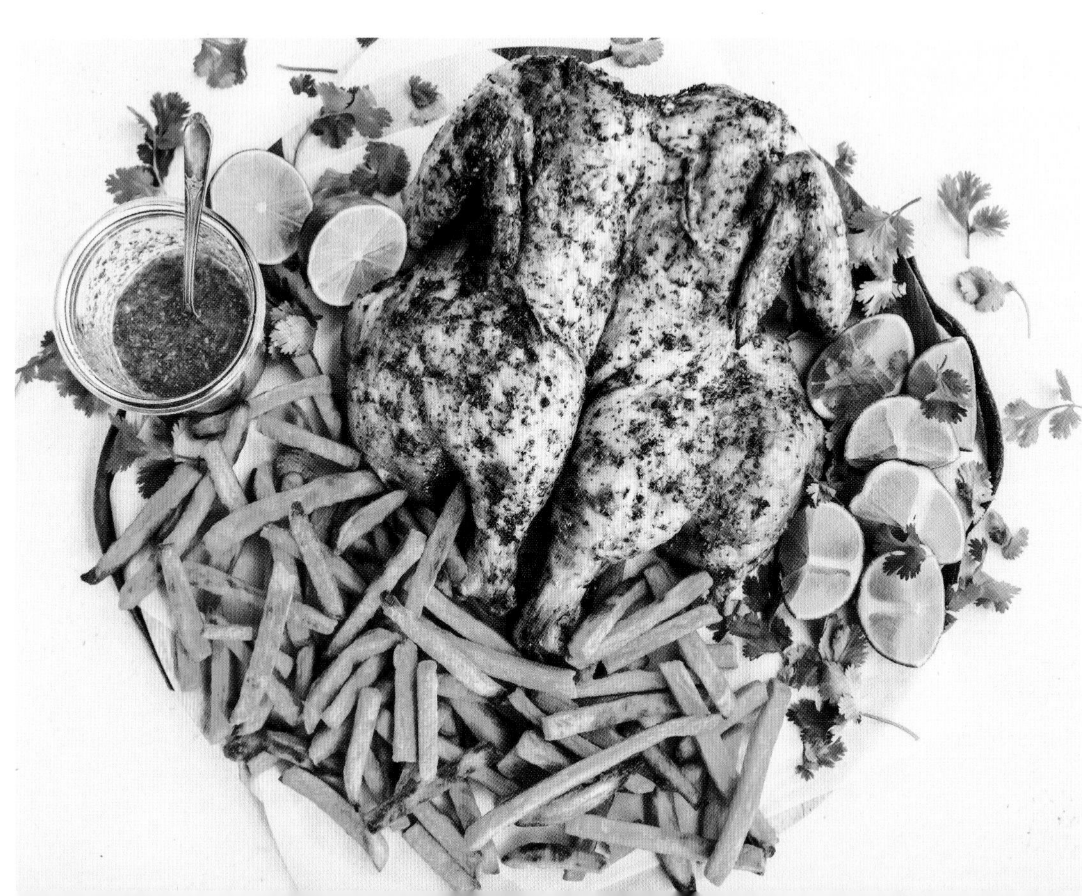

MARINADE AND CHICKEN

1. Preheat the oven to 350°F (180°C or gas mark 4).
2. Place the cilantro, olive oil, lime juice, garlic, salt, pepper, and onion powder in a food processor. Pulse until fully combined.
3. Place the chicken on a cutting board, breast-side down. Use a sharp pair of kitchen shears and cut along both sides of the backbone. Remove the backbone completely. Next, turn the chicken front-side up and flatten it with the heel of your hand. You may need to use the pressure of both hands to flatten completely.
4. Set aside a little bit of the marinade in a small bowl to coat the chicken once it is done cooking. Place the chicken in a large roasting pan, breast-side up, and coat the entire surface of the chicken with the marinade (I use my hands).
5. Bake the chicken for 45 minutes, then increase the oven temperature to 450°F (230°C or gas mark 8). Continue baking until a thermometer inserted into a meaty part of the leg registers 160°F (71°C), about 15 minutes more.
6. Remove the chicken from the oven and let rest for at least 10 minutes before brushing with the reserved marinade and carving.
7. Serve with lime wedges and a side of sweet potato fries.

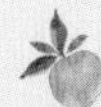

RECIPE NOTES

If you don't want to butterfly the chicken yourself, ask your butcher to do it for you. And if you don't have an air fryer, simply bake the fries while the chicken rests. Toss with the olive oil, salt, garlic powder, and pepper. Bake at 425°F (220°C or gas mark 7) for 20 to 30 minutes, flipping once.

SWEET POTATO FRIES

1. Preheat the air fryer to 400°F (200°C) for 8 minutes.
2. Spray the air fryer basket with olive oil cooking spray.
3. Put the cut fries into a bowl and toss with the olive oil, salt, garlic powder, and pepper.
4. In order to get these good and crispy, place the fries in the basket with space between so they are not touching (you may have to cook in two batches). Spray a little bit of cooking spray on the fries before cooking. Cook the fries for 8 minutes, shaking the basket halfway through cooking.

Crispy Fish Tacos with Pineapple-Broccoli Slaw

These crispy fish tacos are what dreams are made of. Old Bay–seasoned fish sticks are pure bliss when stuffed into butter lettuce and topped with a sweet and crunchy slaw.

SQUEAKY CLEAN PALEO / KETO PALEO / TRADITIONAL PALEO

Makes: 6 to 8 tacos / **Prep Time:** 10 minutes / **Total Time:** 35 minutes

TACOS

- 1 cup (96 g) almond flour
- 3 tablespoons (18 g) arrowroot powder
- 1½ teaspoons Old Bay Seasoning
- ½ teaspoon dried parsley
- ½ teaspoon garlic powder
- ¼ teaspoon sea salt
- ¼ teaspoon black pepper
- 1 large egg
- 1 pound (454 g) firm white fish fillets (such as cod), cut into 1 by 3-inch (2.5 by 7.5 cm) sticks
- 1 head butter lettuce, leaves washed and dried on a paper towel
- ½ cup (120 ml) Ranch Dressing (page 30)

BROCCOLI SLAW

- 2 cups (140 g) packaged broccoli slaw
- ¼ cup (40 g) diced fresh pineapple
- Juice of 1 lime
- 1 tablespoon (15 ml) light olive oil
- ¼ teaspoon sea salt
- Black pepper to taste

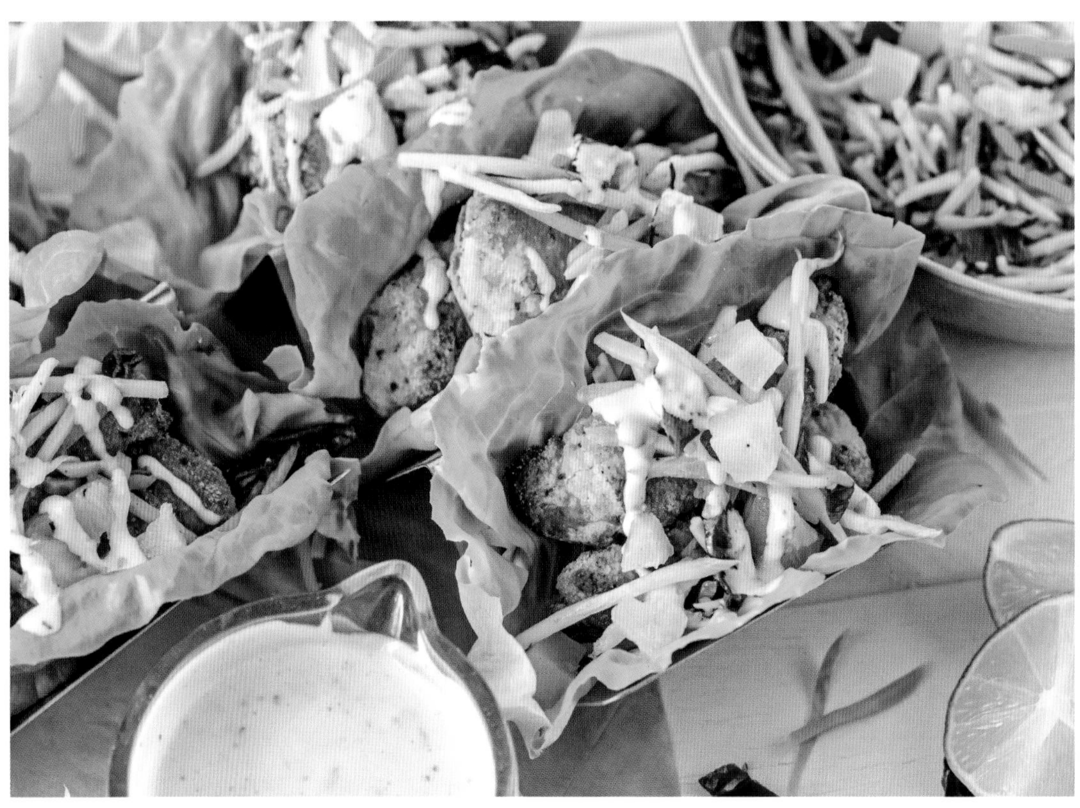

TACOS

1. Preheat the oven to 425°F (220°C or gas mark 7) and coat a baking sheet with olive oil cooking spray.
2. In a medium bowl, whisk together the almond flour, arrowroot, Old Bay, parsley, garlic powder, salt, and pepper.
3. Whisk the egg in a separate medium bowl.
4. With one hand, dip a fish stick into the egg bowl, coating the entire stick, then transfer to the dry bowl with the other hand. Be sure to coat well with the flour. Place on the prepared baking sheet. Repeat until all the sticks are coated.
5. Bake until the fish is cooked and golden brown, flipping over halfway through, 18 to 20 minutes.
6. Assemble the tacos by placing the lettuce cups on a plate and topping each with 2 fish sticks and 1 tablespoon (5 g) broccoli slaw.
7. Drizzle with the ranch before serving.

BROCCOLI SLAW

1. Add the broccoli slaw and pineapple to a medium bowl. Gently toss to combine.
2. In a separate bowl, whisk together the lime juice, olive oil, salt, and pepper.
3. Pour the liquid mixture over the slaw and toss to combine.
4. If there is additional slaw left over, transfer to an airtight storage container and refrigerate for an additional day.

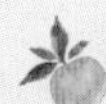

RECIPE NOTES

These tacos also go great with the Mango and Pineapple Salsa on page 57. For Keto, leave out the pineapple and subsitute with ½ avocado, diced.

Burger Bowls

When you get a craving for a big juicy burger, whip up these super-simple keto Paleo burger bowls. Filled with all the traditional toppings of a regular burger—crispy bacon, mustard, tomatoes, red onion, plus an amazing garlic aioli—these are great for quick lunches and on-the-go dinners.

SQUEAKY CLEAN PALEO / KETO PALEO / TRADITIONAL PALEO

Makes: 4 servings / **Prep Time:** 7 minutes / **Total Time:** 20 minutes

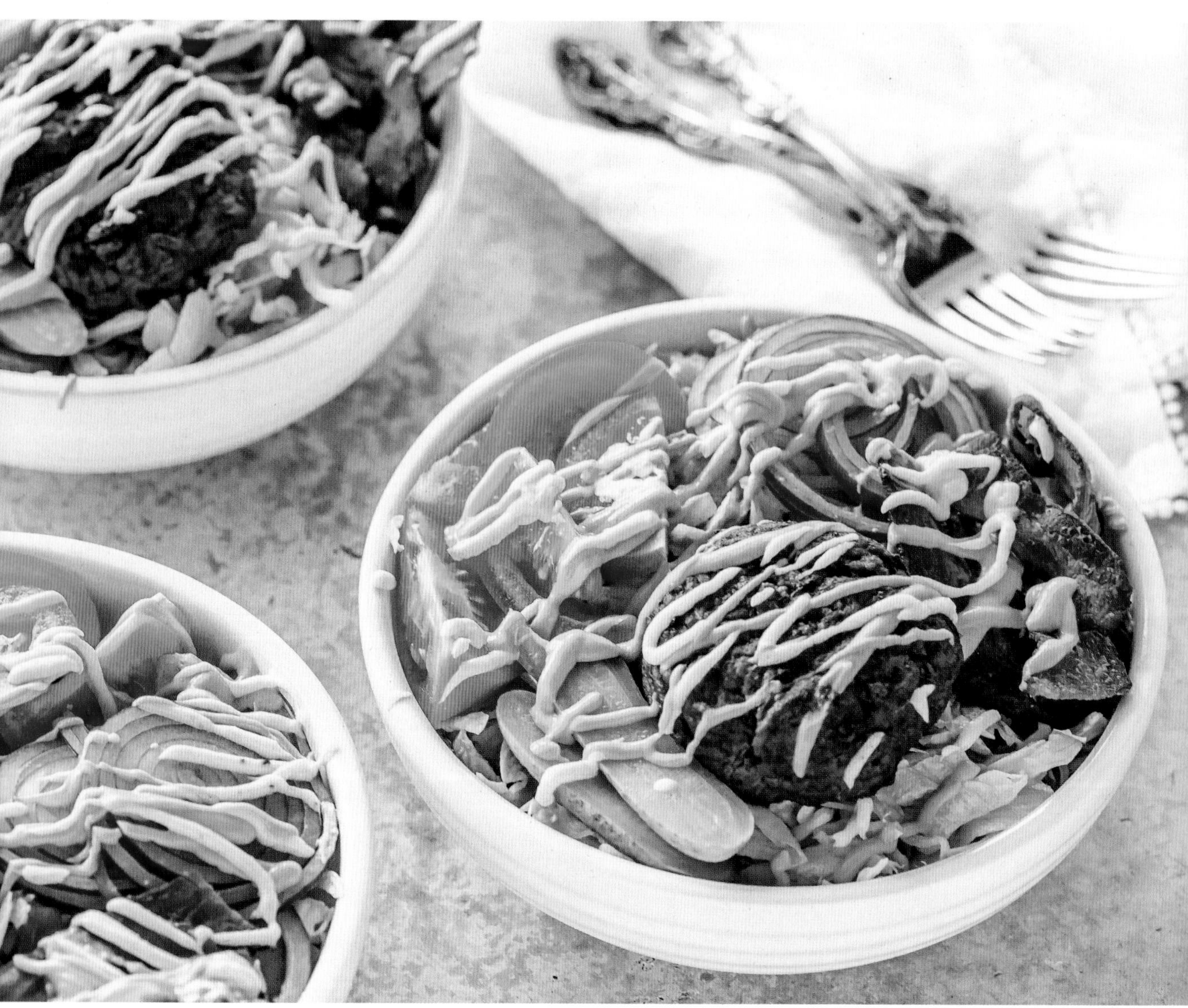

BURGER PATTIES

- 1 pound (454 g) 90/10 ground beef
- ½ teaspoon garlic powder
- ½ teaspoon sea salt
- ¼ teaspoon black pepper
- 1 tablespoon (15 ml) olive oil

BOWLS

- 4 slices compliant bacon
- 8 cups (240 g) shredded iceberg lettuce
- ½ red onion, sliced
- 4 no-sugar-added dill pickles, sliced in half lengthwise
- 4 Roma tomatoes, quartered
- Yellow mustard

GARLIC AIOLI

- 1 cup (240 g) Mayo (page 28) or compliant mayonnaise
- 2 cloves garlic
- 1 teaspoon Dijon mustard
- Sea salt, to taste
- ¼ teaspoon black pepper

BURGER PATTIES

1. In a large bowl, mix together the ground beef, garlic powder, salt, and pepper. Gently form into 4 hamburger patties. Indent the middle of each patty with your thumb to help keep the form while cooking.
2. Heat the olive oil in a large skillet over medium-high heat. Add the patties, leaving space between them.
3. Cook the patties until the desired doneness or when the internal temperature reaches 160°F (71°C), 5 to 6 minutes per side.
4. Once the burgers are cooked, remove to a plate.

BOWLS

1. Preheat the oven to 400°F (200°C or gas mark 6).
2. Place the bacon on a baking sheet and bake until the desired crispiness, 10 to 15 minutes. When cooked, transfer to a plate lined with a paper towel.
3. When the burgers are done, build the burger bowls by adding 2 cups (60 g) lettuce, red onion, 2 dill pickle halves, 4 tomato quarters, and 1 piece of bacon to each of 4 bowls. Top with a burger patty.
4. Squeeze the mustard and Garlic Aioli over the top of each bowl before serving.

GARLIC AIOLI

1. Place the mayo, garlic, mustard, salt, and pepper into a wide-mouth mason jar. Use an immersion blender to blend until combined. Or add to a food processor and blend until smooth. Taste and add more salt and pepper if necessary.
2. Place in a squeeze bottle that has a lid. Will keep in the fridge for up to 1 week.

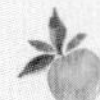

RECIPE NOTES

These tacos also go great with the Mango and Pineapple Salsa on page 57.

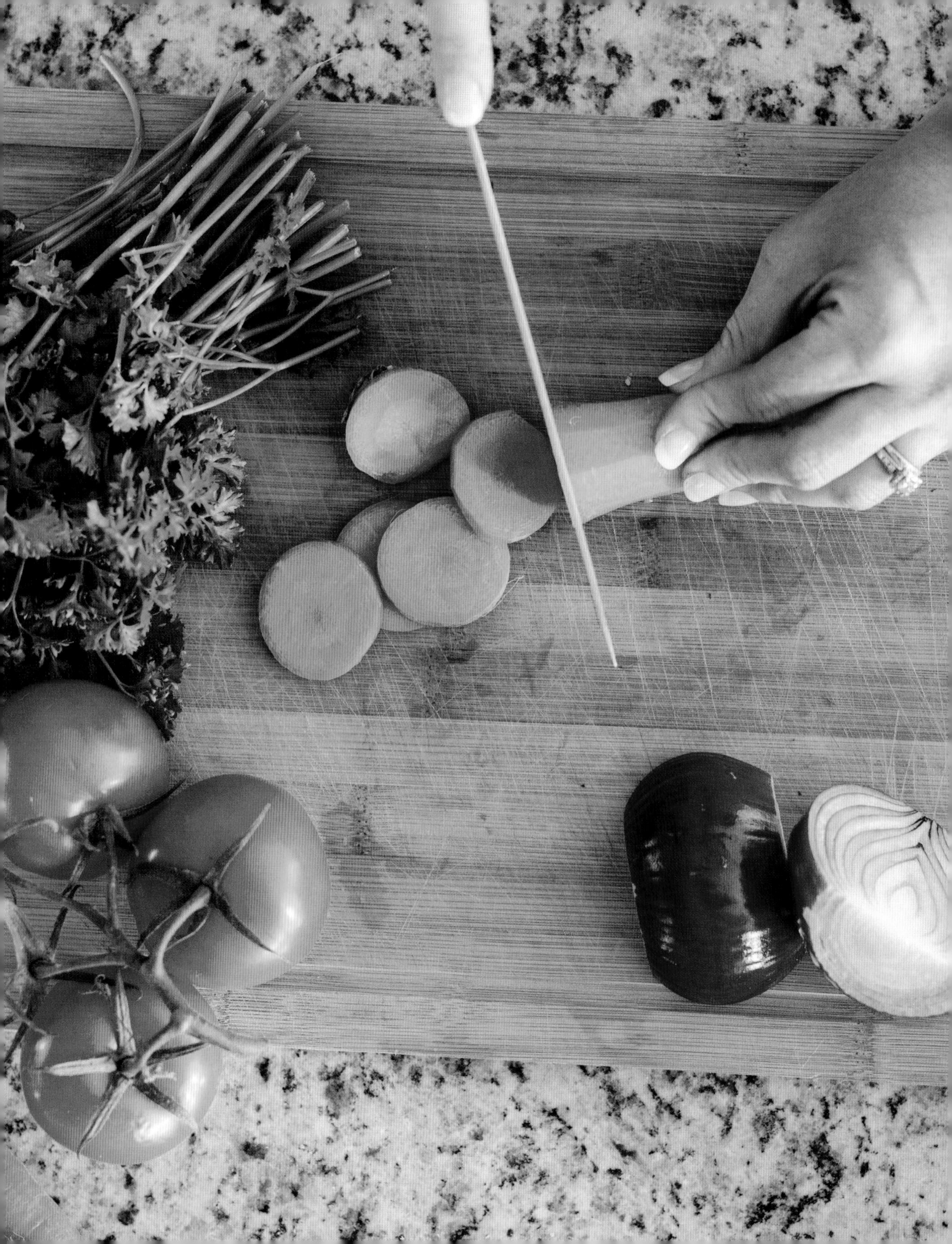

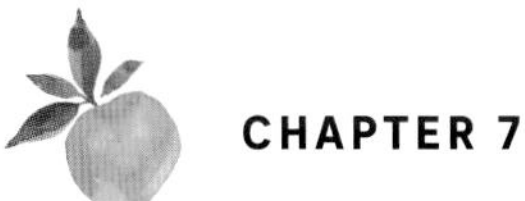

CHAPTER 7

Electric Pressure Cooker and Slow Cooker Meals

Life gets busy sometimes, and there's not enough time to spend it standing in the kitchen playing Martha Stewart. That's when slow cookers and electric pressure cookers save the day. You better believe I will be using my slow cooker daily once fall rolls around! If you are running from place to place and trying to keep up with never-ending ball games or dance lessons, pull out that dang slow cooker (or electric pressure cooker) and make good enough, good enough. If your kids scream for fast food, you look them square in the eyes and say, "Not today, kids . . . Not. Today!"

Beef Tips and Gravy

Hands down, this is one of the best recipes in the entire cookbook. If you want to take Paleo comfort food to a whole new level, put this on the menu tonight. No one will ever guess that this dish is considered healthy. Serve it over Cauliflower Mash (page 96) to change your life!

SQUEAKY CLEAN PALEO / KETO PALEO / TRADITIONAL PALEO

Makes: 4 servings / **Prep Time:** 5 to 10 minutes / **Total Time (Electric Pressure Cooker):** 20 minutes

Total Time (Slow Cooker): 7 to 8 hours / **Total Time (Stove Top):** 25 minutes

SIRLOIN TIPS

1 tablespoon (15 ml) olive oil

2 pounds (910 g) cubed beef stew meat or sirloin tips

½ teaspoon sea salt

Pinch of black pepper

GRAVY

2 cups (480 ml) compliant beef broth (+ 1 cup [240 ml] for slow cooker)

1½ teaspoons ghee

1 teaspoon garlic powder

¼ teaspoon sea salt

¼ teaspoon black pepper

2 tablespoons (12 g) tapioca flour or arrowroot powder dissolved in 2 tablespoons (30 ml) water (see Note)

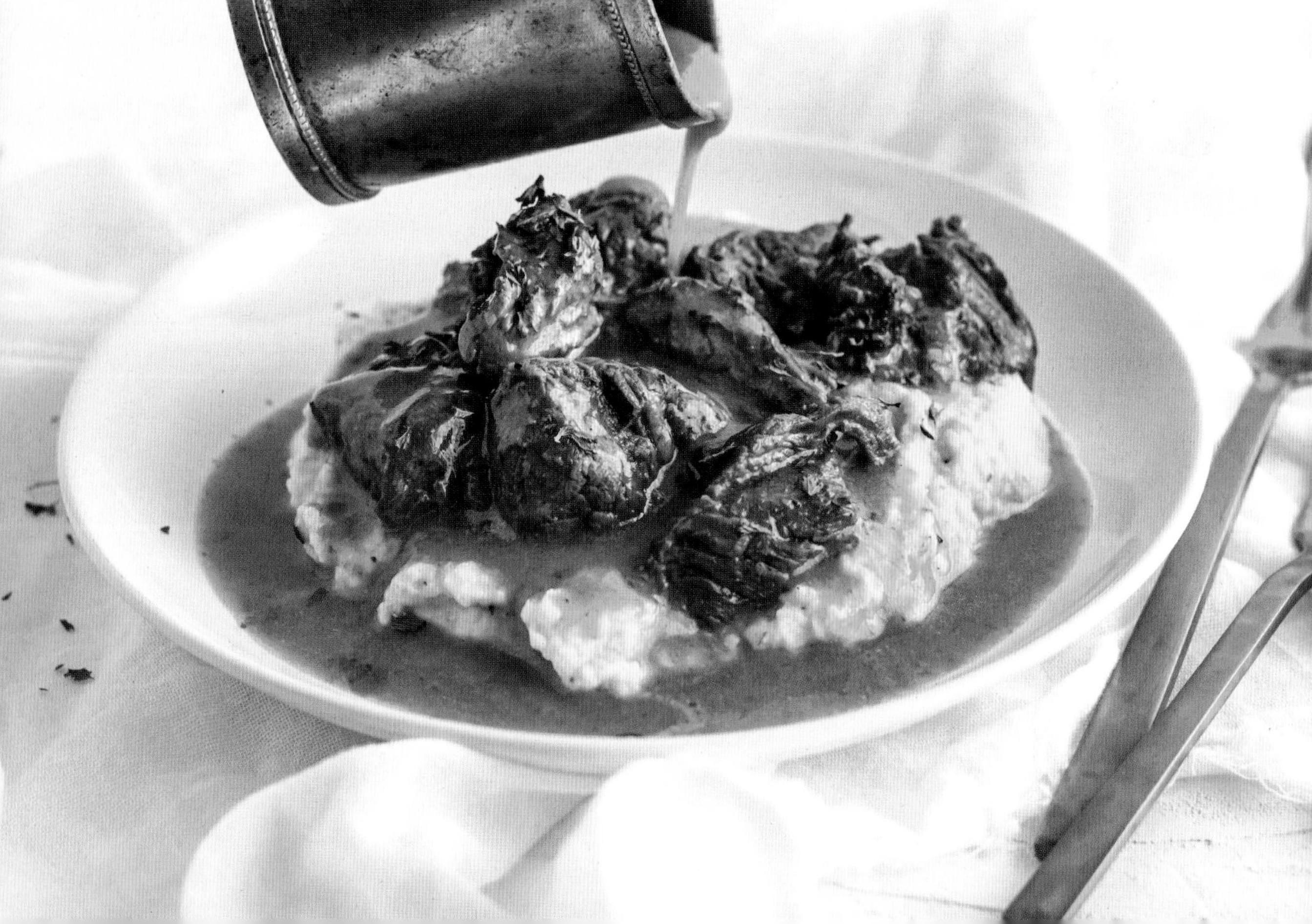

ELECTRIC PRESSURE COOKER VERSION

1. Set the electric pressure cooker to SAUTÉ and allow time for it to heat up. Have all the gravy ingredients ready to go.
2. Add the olive oil to the pot and sprinkle the beef pieces with ½ teaspoon salt and a pinch of black pepper, then place the meat in the pot. Cook, stirring, until the outside of the steak is browned, 4 to 5 minutes.
3. Before adding the gravy ingredients, turn the setting on the pot to HIGH pressure. Once this setting is on, add 2 cups (480 ml) broth, ghee, garlic powder, ¼ teaspoon salt, ¼ teaspoon pepper, and tapioca mixture. (Add the tapioca last; it will mix evenly this way.) Stir until combined. Once it heats up, the gravy should thicken.
4. Lock the lid and seal the top vent.
5. Cook for 10 minutes, then naturally release the steam. If the broth is not thick enough after pressure cooking, whisk in 1 to 2 teaspoons more tapioca flour, turn to SAUTÉ mode, and bring to a boil for a minute or two.

RECIPE NOTES

I usually use natural release, but it's fine to do quick release if you're in a hurry. I find that the steak is a little more tender with the natural release.

To make this Keto Paleo, substitute 1½ tablespoons (14 g) gelatin or ¼ teaspoon xanthan gum, dissolved in water. The gravy won't be as thick as when using regular flour. It is the consistency of a thicker soup. Feel free to add less broth to make it thicker, or experiment with adding a little more tapioca flour. Remember that it will thicken as it simmers.

SLOW COOKER VERSION

1. Heat the olive oil in a large skillet over medium-high. Add the beef, ½ teaspoon salt, and a pinch of black pepper and cook, stirring, until the meat is browned on all sides, about 5 minutes. Transfer the meat to the slow cooker.
2. Add 3 cups (720 ml) broth, ghee, garlic powder, ¼ teaspoon salt, and ¼ teaspoon pepper to the slow cooker.
3. Cover and cook until the meat is tender, on HIGH for 3 to 4 hours or on LOW for 5 to 7 hours.
4. Fifteen minutes before serving, dissolve the tapioca in water and add to the slow cooker. Stir to mix in completely. Replace the lid and cook on LOW for 15 minutes more to allow the sauce to thicken. (If you want it a little thicker, you may need to add 1½ teaspoons more tapioca flour.)

STOVE TOP VERSION

1. Heat the olive oil in a large skillet over medium-high heat. Add the beef, ½ teaspoon salt, and a pinch of pepper and cook until the meat is browned on all sides, about 5 minutes.
2. Pour 2 cups (480 ml) broth over the meat and bring to a boil. Reduce the heat, and add the tapioca mixture, ghee, garlic powder, ¼ teaspoon salt, and ¼ teaspoon pepper. The broth will not thicken automatically; it will thicken as it heats up.
3. Mix thoroughly and cover. Simmer, stirring occasionally, until the meat is tender and the gravy is thick, about 15 minutes. The longer it simmers, the more tender the meat.

Shredded Pork

This easy shredded pork will make you forget about that BBQ joint down the street. The recipe has minimal ingredients but maximum flavor. Make a big batch at the beginning of the week and use it for multiple meals throughout the week (see Note).

SQUEAKY CLEAN PALEO / KETO PALEO / TRADITIONAL PALEO

Makes: 8 to 10 servings / **Prep Time:** 7 minutes / **Total Time (Electric Pressure Cooker):** 45 minutes

Total Time (Slow Cooker): 8 hours

- 4 pounds (1.8 kg) boneless pork shoulder
- 1 teaspoon garlic powder
- 1 teaspoon sea salt
- 1 teaspoon black pepper
- ½ cup (120 ml) water
- Juice of ½ lime (optional)

ELECTRIC PRESSURE COOKER VERSION

1. Slice the pork into 4 equal pieces and sprinkle with the garlic powder, salt, and pepper.
2. Place the water in the bottom of the electric pressure cooker and then add the pork.
3. Lock the lid and seal the top vent. Press MANUAL and set for 45 minutes.
4. Allow the pot to naturally release the steam.
5. Remove the pork to a large cutting board and shred with two forks.
6. Add the pork along with the remaining juices from the pot and the lime juice, if using, to a large serving bowl.
7. Store any leftovers in an airtight container along with the juices. Will keep for up to a week in the fridge.

SLOW COOKER VERSION

1. Place the pork on a cutting board and cover the entire piece with the garlic powder, salt, and pepper.
2. Place the water in the bottom of the slow cooker and then add the pork.
3. Cover and cook until the internal temperature reaches 190°F (88°C), on LOW for 7 to 8 hours.
4. Remove the pork to a large cutting board and shred with two forks.
5. Add the pork along with the remaining juices from the pot and the lime juice, if using, to a large serving bowl.

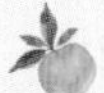

RECIPE NOTES

This dish is great to make in bulk and serve in different ways throughout the week. Check out the following recipes that call for shredded pork: Tostones and Shredded Pork Nachos (page 47), Stuffed Mexican Spaghetti Squash (page 120), and BBQ Ranch Salad (page 81).

Salsa Verde Chicken

Meal prep has never been easier (or yummier) than with this super easy salsa verde chicken. It's so versatile, it can leave you building different delicious meals throughout the week. Add it to a lettuce wrap, on top of salads, or have it with cauliflower rice and veggies.

SQUEAKY CLEAN PALEO / KETO PALEO / TRADITIONAL PALEO

Makes: 6 to 8 servings / **Prep Time:** 5 minutes / **Total Time (Electric Pressure Cooker):** 15 minutes

Total Time (Slow Cooker): 6 to 7 hours

- 2 to 3 teaspoons olive oil
- ½ cup (80 g) chopped yellow onion
- 1 jar (16 ounces [454 g]) compliant, no-sugar-added salsa verde
- 1 can (14 ounces [392 g]) diced tomatoes, drained
- Juice of ½ lime
- 6 chicken breasts (1½ pounds [680 g] total)
- 1 teaspoon ghee
- 1 teaspoon ground cumin
- 1 teaspoon garlic powder
- 1 teaspoon sea salt
- ½ teaspoon black pepper
- ½ teaspoon chili powder

ELECTRIC PRESSURE COOKER VERSION

1. Set the electric pressure cooker to SAUTÉ and allow time for it to heat up.
2. Add 3 teaspoons olive oil and the onion to the pot. Sauté until tender, a minute or two.
3. Add the salsa verde, tomatoes, and lime juice. Stir to combine.
4. Submerge the chicken breasts in the liquid. Add the ghee, cumin, garlic powder, salt, pepper, and chili powder.
5. Lock the lid and seal the top vent.
6. Cook on HIGH pressure for 10 minutes, then quick release the steam until the pin drops.
7. Shred the chicken in the pot using two forks or an electric mixer (see Note).
8. Mix the shredded chicken with the juices in the pot before serving.

SLOW COOKER VERSION

1. Heat a small skillet with 2 teaspoons olive oil over medium-high heat. Add the onion and cook until tender, 3 minutes. Set aside.
2. Place the chicken breasts in the slow cooker.
3. Top with the salsa verde, tomatoes, cooked onion, lime juice, ghee, cumin, garlic powder, salt, pepper, and chili powder.
4. Cover and cook until the chicken is tender, on HIGH for 3 to 4 hours or on LOW for 7 to 8 hours.
5. Shred the chicken in the pot using two forks or an electric mixer (see Note).
6. Mix the shredded chicken with the juices in the pot before serving.

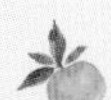

RECIPE NOTES

Store the shredded chicken in the juices in an airtight container in the refrigerator for up to 5 days, or in the freezer for up to 3 months.

Pot Roast and Curry Coleslaw

Pot roast is something I think we can all agree brings true happiness to tummies everywhere. This recipe is so simple, yet it explodes with flavor. Serving this pot roast over my Grandmother Sue Sue's curry coleslaw will change everything you have ever known about a traditional roast.

SQUEAKY CLEAN PALEO / KETO PALEO / TRADITIONAL PALEO

Makes: 4 servings / **Prep Time:** 10 minutes / **Total Time (Electric Pressure Cooker):** 30 minutes

Total Time (Slow Cooker): 7 to 8 hours

POT ROAST

1 tablespoon (15 ml) olive oil (for the electric pressure cooker)
2 pounds (910 g) beef chuck roast
Sea salt and black pepper, to taste
2 cups (480 ml) compliant beef broth
1 sweet onion, cut into big chunks
3 tablespoons (45 ml) compliant hot sauce
2 cloves garlic, coarsely chopped

CURRY COLESLAW

4 cups (280 g) packaged coleslaw mix
½ cup (240 g) Mayo (page 28) or compliant mayonnaise
1 teaspoon curry powder
Sea salt and black pepper, to taste
Splash of rice vinegar

ELECTRIC PRESSURE COOKER VERSION

1. Set the electric pressure cooker to SAUTÉ and allow time for it to heat up. Add the olive oil. Sprinkle the roast with salt and pepper and add it to the pot. Brown on each side, about 4 minutes total.
2. Set the pot to HIGH pressure and add the broth, onion, hot sauce, and garlic.
3. Lock the lid and seal the top vent. Cook until tender, 20 minutes, then naturally release the steam. (If the roast is frozen, cook an additional 10 to 12 minutes.)
4. Use a fork to shred the roast right in the pot (it absorbs any extra juice).
5. Add 1 cup (70 g) of coleslaw to each of 4 bowls and top with the shredded roast and a little bit of broth.

RECIPE NOTES

I usually use natural release, but it's fine to do quick release if you're in a hurry. I find that the meat is a little more tender with the natural release.

SLOW COOKER VERSION

1. Turn the slow cooker on LOW. Add the broth and the roast.
2. Completely cover the top of the roast with the salt, pepper, onion, and garlic.
3. Add the hot sauce to the top of the meat and spices.
4. Cover and cook until the internal temperature reaches 190°F (88°C), on LOW for 6 to 7 hours.
5. Use a fork to shred the roast in the pot.
6. Add 1 cup (70 g) of coleslaw to each of 4 bowls and top with the shredded roast and a little bit of broth.

CURRY COLESLAW

In a medium bowl, add the coleslaw mix, mayo, curry, salt, pepper, and rice vinegar. Use a spoon to mix together until well combined.

RECIPE NOTES

If there are leftovers, put the roast and juices in an airtight container and store for up to 1 week. Store the coleslaw in an airtight container for a day or 2.

Chili

Chili screams tailgating, football, and cold fall or winter nights. If you find yourself craving something to warm your soul during the colder months, or needing a change from all things grilled in the summer, throw this chili on your stove or in your slow cooker.

SQUEAKY CLEAN PALEO / KETO PALEO / TRADITIONAL PALEO

Makes: 8 to 10 servings / **Prep Time:** 10 minutes / **Total Time (Stove Top):** 40 minutes

Total Time (Slow Cooker): 7 to 8 hours

- 1 tablespoon light olive oil
- 2 cloves garlic, minced
- 2 pounds 90/10 ground beef or 85/15 ground turkey
- 3 cans (14.5 ounces) diced tomatoes (petite or regular)
- 1 can (8 ounces) no-sugar-added tomato sauce
- ¾ cup compliant beef broth
- ⅓ cup water
- 3 tablespoons tomato paste
- 1 lime, juiced
- 1 sweet onion, finely chopped
- 2 tablespoons chili powder
- 1½ teaspoons ground cumin
- 1¼ teaspoons garlic powder
- 1 teaspoon crushed red pepper flakes
- 1 teaspoon sea salt
- ½ teaspoon onion powder
- ½ teaspoon black pepper
- ¼ teaspoon cayenne pepper
- 1 avocado, diced
- ⅓ cup chopped cilantro

STOVE TOP VERSION

1. Heat the olive oil in a 5- or 6-quart Dutch oven or soup pot over medium. Add the garlic and cook until fragrant, 1 minute.
2. Add the ground meat and onion and cook until browned, 6 minutes.
3. Add the tomatoes, tomato sauce, broth, water, tomato paste, lime juice, chili powder, cumin, garlic powder, red pepper flakes, salt, onion powder, black pepper, and cayenne pepper. Stir to combine. Bring to a boil, then reduce the heat and simmer for 30 minutes. Taste and add more salt, if desired.
4. Divide among bowls and garnish with the avocado and cilantro before serving.

SLOW COOKER VERSION

1. Heat the olive oil in a large skillet over medium-high. Add the ground beef, onion, and garlic. Cook until the meat is browned and the onion is translucent, 6 minutes.
2. Transfer to the slow cooker. Add the tomatoes, tomato sauce, broth, water, tomato paste, lime juice, chili powder, cumin, garlic powder, red pepper flakes, salt, onion salt, black pepper, and cayenne pepper. Stir to combine.
3. Cover and cook on LOW for 6 to 8 hours.
4. Divide among bowls and garnish with the avocado and cilantro before serving.

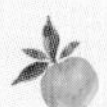

RECIPE NOTES

Enjoy this chili in a bowl or make a big batch and serve it different ways throughout the week. Stuff it in a sweet potato or pour over plantain chips or tostones for easy nachos. For kids, pour it over clean, nitrate-free hot dogs. If there's any extra, store it in an airtight container in the refrigerator for up to 1 week or in the freezer for 3 to 4 months.

Cabbage Roll Soup

This Paleo cabbage roll soup screams comfort food—and it's so much easier than making a batch of traditional cabbage rolls. Throw all the ingredients into the crockpot and simmer all day for an easy weeknight or weekend lunch or dinner that the whole family will love.

SQUEAKY CLEAN PALEO / KETO PALEO / TRADITIONAL PALEO

Makes: 8 servings / **Prep Time:** 10 minutes / **Total Time (Stove Top):** 40 minutes

Total Time (Slow Cooker): 7 to 8 hours

1 tablespoon olive oil
1 yellow onion, chopped
3 cloves garlic, minced
1 pound (450 g) 90/10 ground beef
1 pound (450 g) no sugar added sausage
5 cups compliant beef broth
5 cups coarsely chopped cabbage (about ½ medium head)
1 can (28 ounces) diced tomatoes, undrained
1 can (8 ounces) no-sugar-added tomato sauce
½ cup (120 ml) water
2 tablespoons tomato paste
1 teaspoon coconut aminos
1 teaspoon paprika
1 teaspoon dried oregano
1 teaspoon dried basil
1 teaspoon sea salt
½ teaspoon onion powder
½ teaspoon black pepper
Fresh chopped parsley, for garnish

STOVE TOP VERSION

1. Heat the olive oil in a 5- or 6-quart Dutch oven or large pot over medium-high. Add the onion and garlic and cook until translucent, 2 minutes. Add the beef and sausage and cook until brown, 4 to 5 minutes.
2. Add the broth, cabbage, tomatoes (with liquid), tomato sauce, water, tomato paste, coconut aminos, paprika, oregano, basil, salt, onion powder, and pepper. Stir to combine.
3. Bring to a boil, then reduce the heat and simmer until the cabbage is very tender, 30 minutes.
4. Divide among bowls and garnish with the parsley before serving.

SLOW COOKER VERSION

1. Heat the olive oil in a large skillet over medium-high. Add the tablespoon olive oil and the ground beef and sausage along with the garlic and onion. Cook until the meat is browned and onion is translucent, 2 minutes.
2. Transfer to the slow cooker. Add the broth, cabbage, tomatoes (with liquid), tomato sauce, water, tomato paste, coconut aminos, paprika, oregano, basil, salt, onion powder, and pepper. Stir to combine.
3. Cover and cook on LOW for 6 to 8 hours.
4. Divide among bowls and garnish with the parsley before serving.

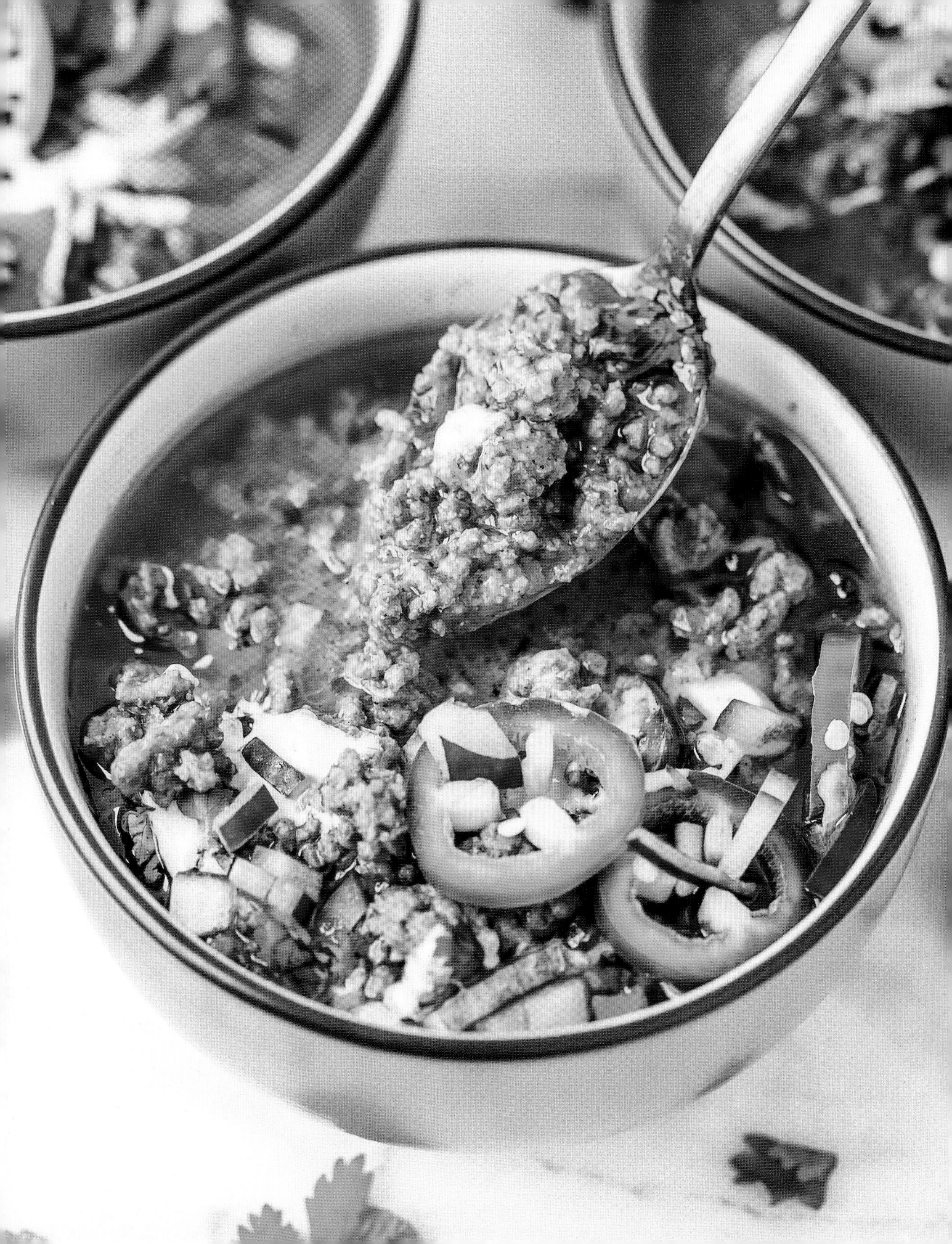

Taco Soup

Taco Tuesday has never looked so good! Give your traditional tacos a facelift with this easy soup that is perfect for any time of the year. Want to really impress your family with leftovers? Reinvent this soup into another meal during the week by throwing a cup of it in a baked sweet potato. Pretty genius, huh?

SQUEAKY CLEAN PALEO / KETO PALEO / TRADITIONAL PALEO

Makes: 8 servings / **Prep Time:** 10 minutes / **Total Time (Stove Top):** 40 minutes

Total Time (Slow Cooker): 7 to 8 hours

1 tablespoon (15 ml) olive oil
½ sweet onion, finely chopped
1 clove garlic, minced
2 pounds 90/10 ground beef
6 cups compliant beef broth
1 can (14.5 ounces) crushed tomatoes
1 can (8 ounces) no-sugar-added tomato sauce
½ cup (120 ml) water
½ lime, juiced
1½ tablespoons chili powder
2 teaspoons ground cumin
1 teaspoon paprika
1 teaspoon dried oregano
1 teaspoon black pepper
1 teaspoon ghee
½ teaspoon garlic powder
½ teaspoon onion powder
½ teaspoon sea salt
For garnish: fresh sliced jalapeños, fresh chopped cilantro, red onion, Ranch Dressing (page 30), lime wedges

STOVE TOP VERSION

1. Heat the oil in a 5- or 6-quart Dutch oven or soup pot over medium. Add the onion and garlic.
2. Add the ground beef and cook until the meat is browned and the onion is translucent, 2 to 3 minutes.
3. Add the broth, tomatoes, tomato sauce, water, lime juice, chili powder, cumin, paprika, oregano, pepper, ghee, garlic powder, onion powder, and salt. Stir to combine.
4. Bring to a boil, then reduce the heat and simmer for 30 minutes.
5. Divide among bowls and garnish with jalapeños, cilantro, red onion, homemade ranch, and lime wedges, as desired.

SLOW COOKER VERSION

1. Heat the oil in a large skillet over medium-high. Add the onion, garlic, and ground beef. Cook until the meat is browned and the onion is translucent, 6 minutes.
2. Transfer to the slow cooker. Add the broth, tomatoes, tomato sauce, water, lime juice, chili powder, cumin, paprika, oregano, pepper, ghee, garlic powder, onion powder, and salt. Stir to combine.
3. Cover and cook on LOW for 6 to 8 hours.
4. Divide among bowls and garnish with lime juice, jalapeños, cilantro, red onion, and homemade ranch as desired.

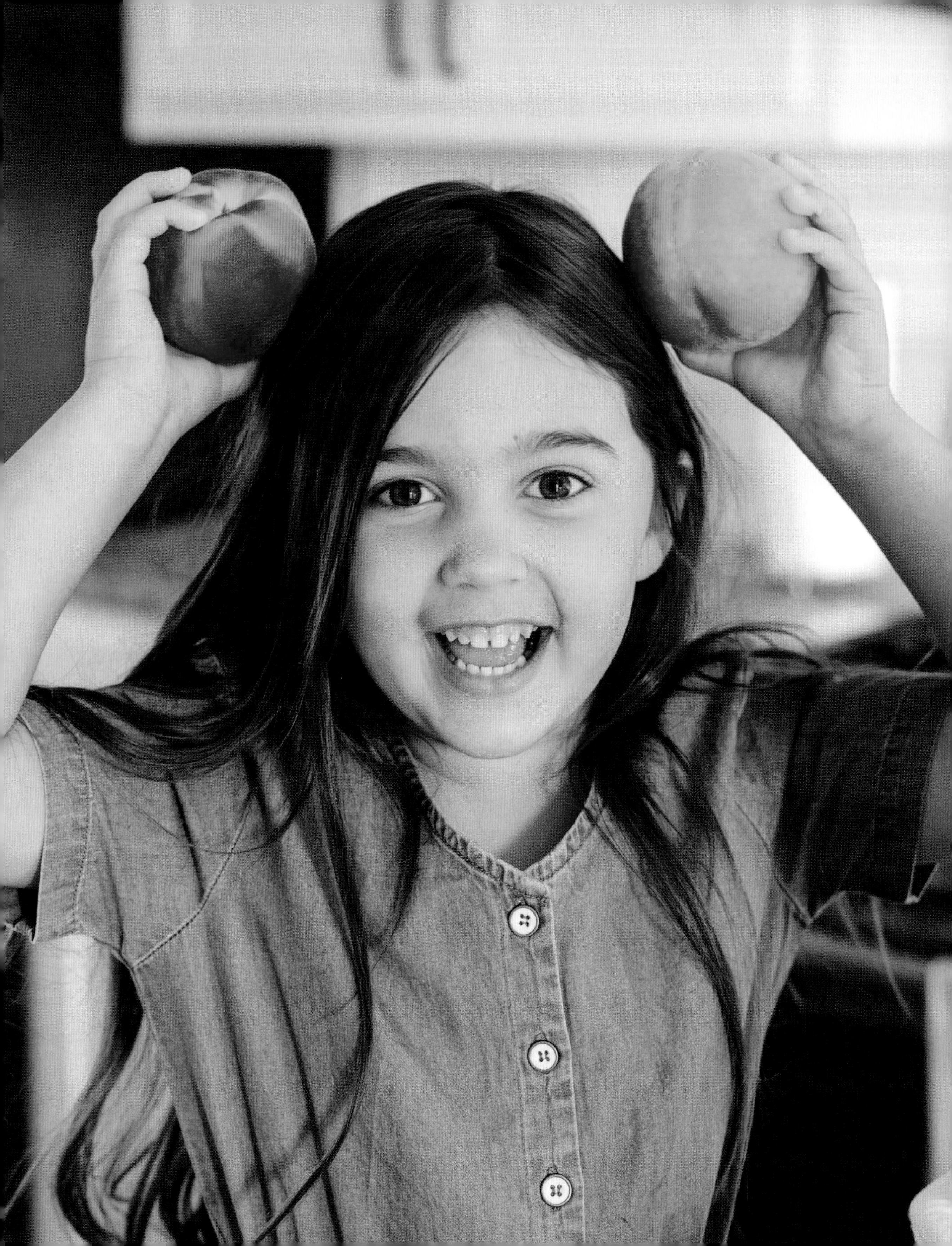

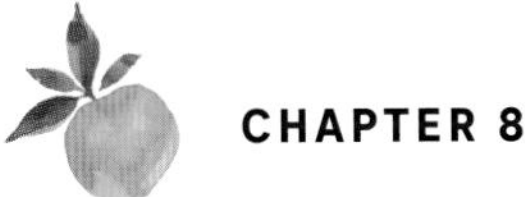

CHAPTER 8

Kid-Approved Dishes

I love when my girls come running to the table when I scream, "Dinnertime!" For me, as a mom, it's super important to build beautiful memories with healthy yet craveable meals. All the recipes found in this section are kid approved and will keep your sweet children reaching for more. Be careful, though: Adults can easily get hooked on these recipes. Grown-ups are never too old to be kids . . . right?

Turkey Meatloaf Muffins

Want your kids to give you two thumbs up for dinner tonight? These meatloaf muffins are so simple and versatile—and they're perfectly sized for little hands. Serve them for dinner or even as easy grab-and-go lunchbox or snack options throughout the week. You can also make a big batch to freeze. If stored in an airtight freezer-proof container, they will keep for up to 2 months.

SQUEAKY CLEAN PALEO / KETO PALEO / TRADITIONAL PALEO

Makes: 12 muffins / **Prep Time:** 10 minutes / **Total Time:** 30 to 35 minutes

---

1 tablespoon (15 ml) olive oil
½ cup (80 g) chopped sweet onion
1 clove garlic, minced
2 pounds (910 g) ground turkey
½ cup (48 g) almond flour
1 egg, beaten
1 teaspoon coconut aminos
1 teaspoon dried oregano
1 teaspoon sea salt
¼ teaspoon black pepper
1 cup (240 g) Ketchup (recipe follows) or compliant ketchup, divided

---

1. Preheat the oven to 350°F (180°C or gas mark 4) and coat a 12-cup muffin tin with olive oil cooking spray.
2. Heat the olive oil in a small skillet over medium-high heat. Add the onion and garlic and cook until translucent, 2 minutes. Remove from the heat and set aside.
3. In a large mixing bowl, add the ground turkey, almond flour, egg, coconut aminos, oregano, salt, pepper, and ½ cup (120 g) of the ketchup.
4. Transfer the onion and garlic mixture to the turkey bowl and mix together until well combined.
5. Divide the meat mixture among the muffin cups and press down to flatten. Bake for 20 minutes.
6. Remove the muffin tin from the oven and top the muffins with the remaining ½ cup (120 g) ketchup.
7. Return the muffin tin to the oven and bake until the muffins are sizzling and register 160°F (71°C), 10 minutes more.
8. Serve immediately or allow to cool before refrigerating in an airtight container.

KETCHUP

1 can (6 ounces [168 g]) tomato paste
½ cup (120 ml) water (see Note)
3½ tablespoons (52 ml) no-sugar-added tomato sauce
2½ tablespoons (37 ml) apple cider vinegar
2½ tablespoons (37 ml) sweetener of choice (see Note)
1½ tablespoons (23 ml) coconut aminos
½ teaspoon sea salt
½ teaspoon onion powder
½ teaspoon garlic powder
⅛ teaspoon dried mustard powder
⅛ teaspoon ground allspice
Pinch of black pepper

1. In a small saucepan, mix together the tomato paste, water, tomato sauce, vinegar, sweetener, coconut aminos, salt, onion powder, garlic powder, mustard, allspice, and pepper. Bring to a boil.
2. Lower the heat and simmer, stirring occasionally, for about 5 minutes. Taste and add more salt, if needed.
3. Remove from the heat and blend together with an immersion blender or in a high-speed blender for 15 seconds.
4. Allow to cool before transferring to a glass jar. Ketchup will keep in the fridge for up to 3 weeks.

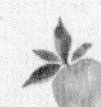

RECIPE NOTES

If you want a thicker or thinner ketchup, simply adjust the amount of water. More water will make it thinner while less will make it thicker. For Squeaky Clean Paleo, substitute 2 pitted dates soaked in hot water for 10 minutes for the sweetener. Simply drain and add the dates in step 3. For Keto Paleo, substitute monk fruit or Paleo maple syrup for the sweetener or omit sweetener altogether. For Traditional Paleo, use any sweetener from the list on page 15.

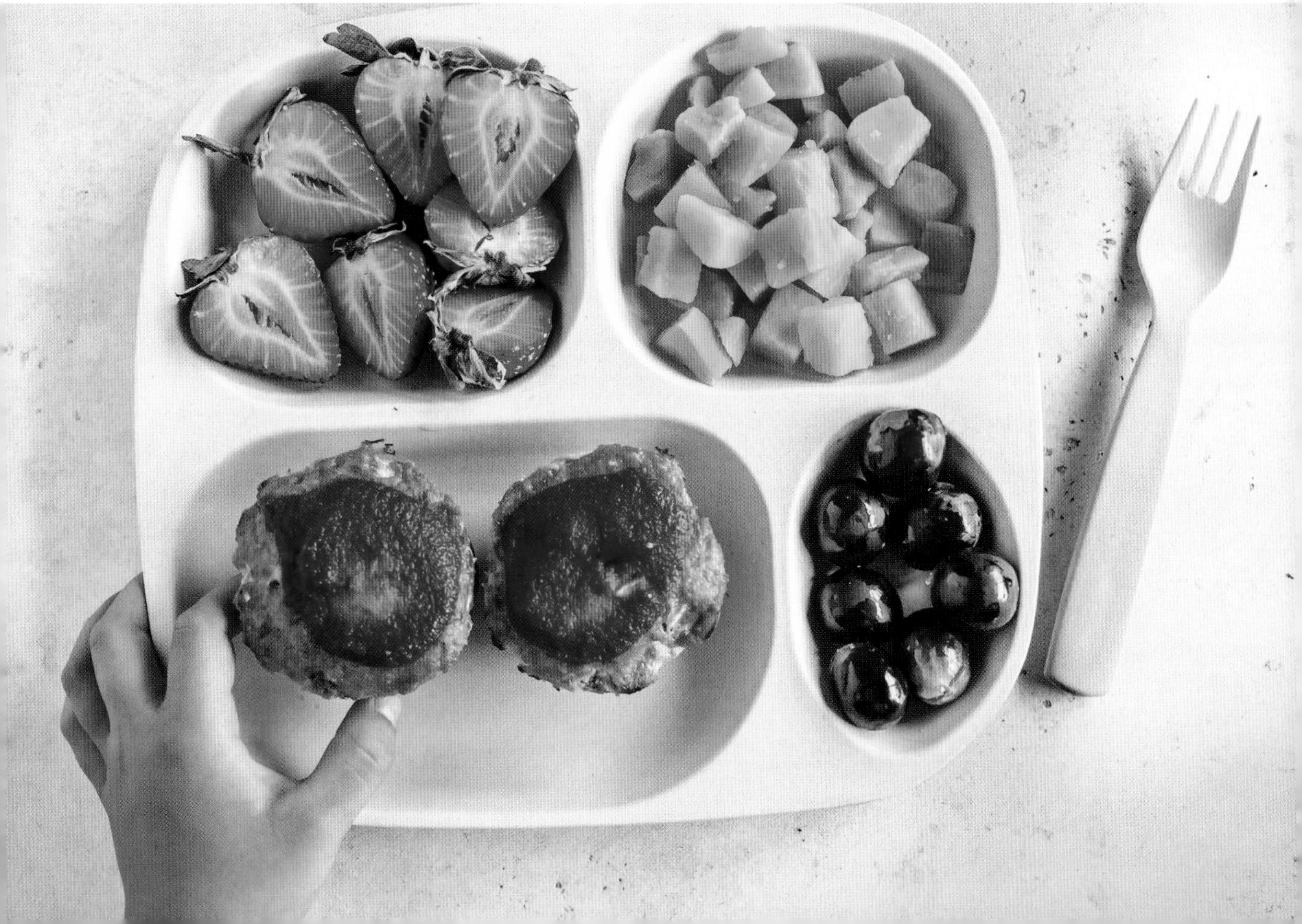

Crispy Chicken Strips

No need to serve your kiddos overprocessed chicken tenders from the freezer anymore. These crispy and crunchy chicken strips will easily become a weekly staple on your kids' dinner plate, along with some roasted veggies.

SQUEAKY CLEAN PALEO / KETO PALEO / TRADITIONAL PALEO

Makes: 4 servings / **Prep Time:** 5 to 10 minutes / **Total Time:** 35 minutes

1 cup (96 g) almond flour
3 tablespoons (18 g) tapioca or coconut flour
1½ tablespoons (6 g) nutritional yeast (optional)
1½ teaspoons sea salt
1½ teaspoons black pepper
½ teaspoon garlic powder
1 large egg
1 pound (454 g) chicken breast tenders
BBQ Sauce (page 35), or Ranch Dressing (page 30), for dipping

OVEN VERSION

1. Preheat the oven to 450°F (230°C or gas mark 8). Line a baking sheet with parchment paper.
2. In a medium bowl, whisk together the almond flour, tapioca flour, nutritional yeast (if using), salt, pepper, and garlic powder.
3. In a separate bowl, whisk the egg.
4. Coat each chicken tender in the egg mixture. Roll in the almond flour mixture, coating thoroughly, and place on the prepared baking sheet.
5. Bake for 12 minutes, then flip, and bake until golden brown, 12 minutes more.
6. Serve with the dipping sauce of choice.

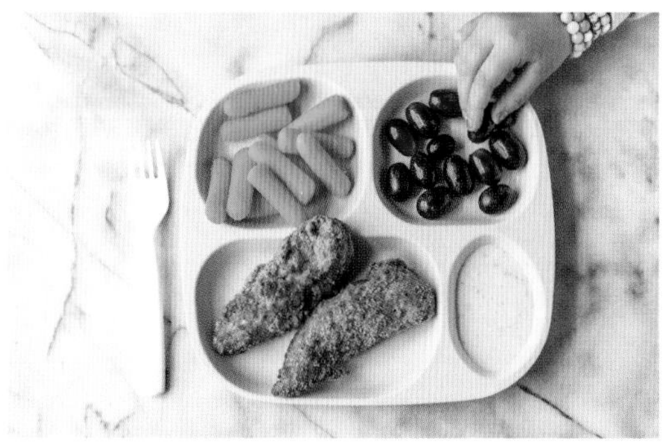

AIR FRYER VERSION

1. Preheat the air fryer to 370°F (188°C). Spray the air fryer basket with olive oil cooking spray.
2. In a medium bowl, whisk together the almond flour, tapioca flour, nutritional yeast (if using), salt, pepper, and garlic powder.
3. In a separate bowl, whisk the egg.
4. Coat each chicken tender in the egg mixture. Roll in the almond flour mixture, coating thoroughly.
5. Place half the chicken tenders in the air fryer basket. Make sure they're not touching; air will need to flow between them as they cook. You will cook two separate batches.
6. Spray a little of the cooking spray on top of each tender and turn the timer on for 12 minutes. Halfway through, pause cooking, flip the tenders, spray the other side with cooking spray, and finish cooking. They should be golden brown with an internal temperature of 160°F (71°C). Repeat this step until all the tenders are cooked.
7. Remove from the air fryer to a serving platter or plate. Serve with the dipping sauce of choice.

Spaghetti Squash and Meat Sauce

Here is a super-simple take on the traditional spaghetti and meat sauce. When you dress up shredded spaghetti squash noodles with a savory meat sauce, you will fool everyone at the table with this healthy, yet comforting, Paleo recipe.

SQUEAKY CLEAN PALEO / TRADITIONAL PALEO

Makes: 6 servings / **Prep Time:** 5 to 10 minutes / **Total Time:** 30 minutes + time to cook the squash

SPAGHETTI SQUASH

1 medium spaghetti squash (4 pounds [1.8 kg])
2 tablespoons (30 ml) olive oil, divided
¼ teaspoon sea salt
¼ teaspoon black pepper

MEAT SAUCE

1 tablespoon (15 ml) olive oil
3 cloves garlic, 1 minced, 2 whole
1 pound (454 g) 90/10 ground beef
2 cans (28 ounces [784 g]) whole peeled tomatoes
2 tablespoons (30 g) tomato paste
1 tablespoon (2 g) dried oregano
1 tablespoon (2 g) dried basil
2 teaspoons dried parsley
½ teaspoon sea salt
¼ teaspoon onion powder
¼ teaspoon black pepper
Nutritional yeast, for garnish (optional)

COOKING SPAGHETTI SQUASH IN THE OVEN

Heat the oven to 400°F (200°C or gas mark 6). Slice the squash in half lengthwise and scoop out the seeds. Drizzle the halves with olive oil and sprinkle with sea salt and pepper. Place cut-side down on a baking sheet and roast until tender, 45 to 50 minutes. Let cool slightly, then use a fork to shred the squash flesh.

COOKING SPAGHETTI SQUASH IN THE ELECTRIC PRESSURE COOKER

Pierce the squash all over with a paring knife. Place a trivet or steamer basket in the bottom of the electric pressure cooker, set the squash on top, and add 1 cup (240 ml) water to the bottom. Cook on high pressure for 15 minutes. Use instant release to release the cooker's pressure. Remove the squash and let cool slightly. Halve lengthwise, drizzle with olive oil, and sprinkle with the salt and pepper. Shred the squash flesh with a fork.

MEAT SAUCE

1. Heat 1 tablespoon (15 ml) olive oil and the minced garlic in a large nonstick skillet over medium-high heat.
2. Add the beef and cook until browned, 5 to 6 minutes. Drain and set aside.
3. Meanwhile, add the tomatoes (with their liquid), tomato paste, and the whole garlic cloves to a blender or food processor and puree until smooth.
4. Place a 5- or 6-quart (4.5 or 5.4 L) Dutch oven or large pot over medium heat. Add the pureed tomato mixture along with the ground beef, oregano, basil, parsley, salt, onion powder, and pepper. Stir until well combined.
5. Bring to a simmer, then lower the heat and simmer, uncovered, until the flavors blend, 20 to 25 minutes, stirring occasionally. Taste and add more salt, if needed.
6. Divide the spaghetti squash among 6 plates and top with the meat sauce. Garnish with a few shakes of nutritional yeast for a cheesy texture and flavor, if desired.

Sloppy Joe Sweet Potato Subs

Kid life just wouldn't be complete without a messy and delicious Sloppy Joe. Take your weeknight dinner up a notch with these healthy and saucy Paleo subs.

SQUEAKY CLEAN PALEO / TRADITIONAL PALEO

Makes: 6 servings / **Prep Time:** 10 minutes / **Total Time:** 25 minutes

---

SWEET POTATO SLICES

2 large sweet potatoes (unpeeled), sliced lengthwise ½ inch (1.3 cm) thick

MEAT MIXTURE

1 tablespoon (15 ml) olive oil
1 medium shallot, chopped, or ¼ cup (40 g) chopped yellow onion
⅓ cup (50 g) chopped green bell pepper
3 tablespoons (27 g) chopped red bell pepper
¼ cup (30 g) chopped carrot
2 small cloves garlic, minced
1 pound (454 g) 90/10 ground beef or 85/15 ground turkey

SAUCE

1 can (8 ounces [224 g]) no-sugar-added tomato sauce
⅓ cup (80 ml) water
2 tablespoons (30 ml) apple cider vinegar
2 large pitted dates, soaked in hot water for 10 minutes
1 tablespoon (15 ml) coconut aminos
2 teaspoons tomato paste
1 teaspoon yellow mustard
1 teaspoon chili powder
½ teaspoon ground cumin
½ teaspoon sea salt
¼ teaspoon black pepper

SWEET POTATO SLICES AND ASSEMBLY

1. Preheat the oven to 400°F (200°C or gas mark 6) and line a baking sheet with parchment paper.
2. Place the sweet potato slices in a single layer on the prepared baking sheet. Bake until the potatoes are tender, 20 minutes.
3. Meanwhile, prepare the meat mixture.
4. Assemble the subs by placing a cooked potato slice on a plate and then covering with the Sloppy Joe mixture. Top with another sweet potato slice.

MEAT MIXTURE

1. While the potato slices are baking, heat the olive oil in a large skillet over medium-high heat. Add the shallot, bell peppers, carrot, and garlic. Cook, stirring occasionally, until the veggies are tender, 4 to 5 minutes.
2. Add the ground beef and crumble the mixture together with a spoon. Cook until the meat is browned, 5 to 6 minutes.
3. Meanwhile, make the sauce.
4. Decrease the heat to low and pour the blended sauce over the beef mixture. Simmer for 5 to 6 minutes to warm through.

SAUCE

In a high-speed blender, add the tomato sauce, water, vinegar, drained dates, coconut aminos, tomato paste, mustard, chili powder, cumin, salt, and pepper. Blend on high speed until smooth.

Pizza Meatballs

Friday nights are for pizza and snuggles. That doesn't mean you have to call in unhealthy delivery. Be mom or dad of the year and whip up these savory pizza meatballs that are sure to please and amaze any crowd.

SQUEAKY CLEAN PALEO / KETO PALEO / TRADITIONAL PALEO

Makes: 18 to 20 meatballs / **Prep Time:** 10 minutes / **Total Time:** 35 minutes

MEATBALLS

2 pounds (910 g) ground beef, turkey, or chicken
1½ cups (360 ml) Pizza Sauce (recipe follows) or compliant pizza sauce, divided
½ cup (50 g) chopped clean pepperoni (optional; see Note)
1 large egg, beaten
3 tablespoons (30 g) chopped sweet onion
2½ tablespoons (15 g) almond flour
1 tablespoon (2 g) dried oregano
1 teaspoon garlic powder
1 teaspoon black pepper
½ teaspoon onion powder
½ teaspoon sea salt

PIZZA SAUCE

1 can (15 ounces [420 g]) no-sugar-added tomato sauce
1 can (6 ounces [168 g]) tomato paste
2 tablespoons (30 ml) water
1 teaspoon dried oregano
1 teaspoon Italian seasoning
½ teaspoon sea salt
½ teaspoon dried basil
½ teaspoon onion powder
½ teaspoon garlic powder
¼ teaspoon black pepper

MEATBALLS

1. Preheat the oven to 400°F (200°C or gas mark 6) and line a baking sheet with parchment paper.
2. In a large mixing bowl, combine the ground beef, 1¼ cups (300 ml) of the pizza sauce, pepperoni (if using), egg, onion, almond flour, oregano, garlic powder, pepper, onion powder, and salt. Mix until everything is completely combined.
3. Use a cookie scoop or a big spoon to scoop the meat and shape into meatballs (about 1½ inches [3.8 cm]) in diameter.
4. Place each meatball 1 inch (2.5 cm) apart on the prepared baking sheet.
5. Bake until the internal temperature reaches 160°F (71°C), 22 to 25 minutes.
6. Use the remaining ¼ cup (60 ml) pizza sauce for dipping.

PIZZA SAUCE

1. In a medium saucepan over medium-high heat, combine the tomato sauce, tomato paste, water, oregano, Italian seasoning, salt, basil, onion powder, garlic powder, and pepper.
2. Bring to a boil, then turn the heat to low. Simmer until the flavors blend and the sauce thickens, 20 minutes.
3. Use immediately or store in the fridge for up to 1 week.

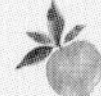

RECIPE NOTES

For Squeaky Clean Paleo, omit the pepperoni. If your meatball mixture is too wet, feel free to add more almond flour.

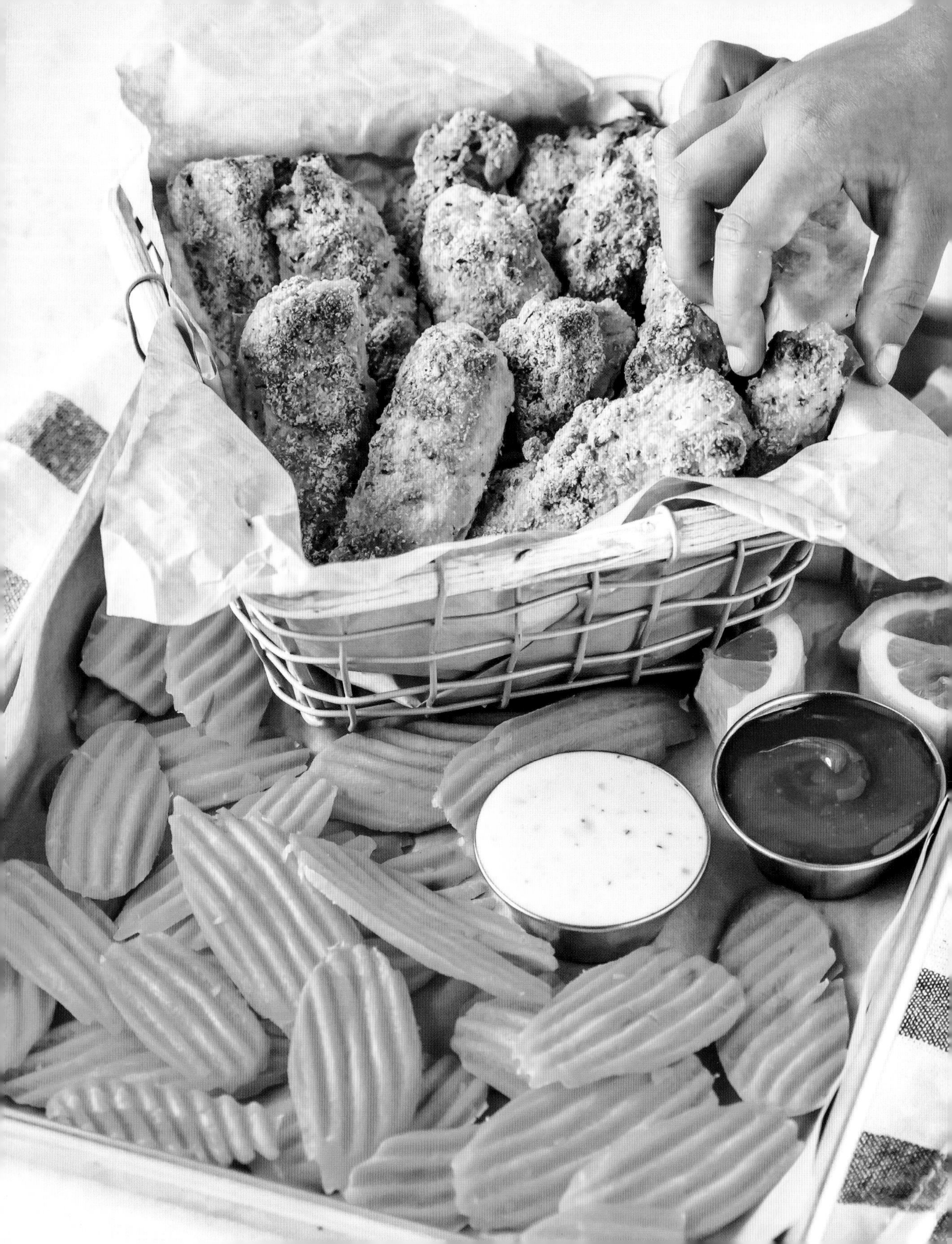

Oven-Baked Fish Sticks

Bring to life your kid's dinner plate with these crunchy, oven-baked fish sticks. Dip them in homemade ranch or ketchup and serve with a side of carrot slices.

SQUEAKY CLEAN PALEO / KETO PALEO / TRADITIONAL PALEO

Makes: About 12 fish sticks / **Prep Time:** 10 minutes / **Total Time:** 35 minutes

---

1 cup (96 g) almond flour
3 tablespoons (18 g) arrowroot flour
1 teaspoon sea salt
½ teaspoon black pepper
½ teaspoon dried parsley
½ teaspoon onion powder
½ teaspoon garlic powder
1 large egg
1 pound (454 g) firm white fish (such as cod), cut into 1 by 3-inch (2.5 by 7.5 cm) sticks
Paleo Ketchup (page 152) or Ranch Dressing (page 30), for serving

---

1. Preheat the oven to 425°F (220°C or gas mark 7) and coat a baking sheet with olive oil cooking spray.
2. In a medium bowl, whisk together the almond flour, arrowroot, salt, pepper, parsley, onion powder, and garlic powder.
3. Whisk the egg in a separate medium bowl.
4. With one hand, dip a fish sticks into the egg bowl and then transfer to the almond flour bowl with the other hand, making sure to evenly coat. Place the fish sticks on the prepared baking sheet. Repeat until all the sticks are coated.
5. Bake until the fish is cooked through and golden brown, flipping over halfway through, 18 to 20 minutes.
6. Serve with your choice of dipping sauce.

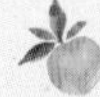

RECIPE NOTES

For Keto, substitute 3 tablespoons coconut flour for the arrowroot flour.

Pancake and Sausage Sliders

Take your kid's breakfast game to the next level with these cute little pancake and sausage sliders. They're perfect topped with fresh fruit and drizzled with maple syrup. Heck, they'll even work as breakfast for dinner!

TRADITIONAL PALEO

Makes: 6 or 7 sliders / **Prep Time:** 10 minutes / **Total Time:** 25 minutes

1 cup (96 g) almond flour
⅓ cup (32 g) arrowroot powder
3 tablespoons (18 g) coconut flour
1 teaspoon baking soda + 1 teaspoon cream of tartar
Pinch of sea salt
½ cup (120 ml) unsweetened almond milk
2 eggs
¼ cup (60 ml) melted ghee
1½ tablespoons (30 g) honey
1 teaspoon vanilla extract
1 pound (454 g) compliant ground sausage
1 tablespoon (15 ml) olive oil
1 cup (150 g) mixed berries (sliced strawberries, blueberries, blackberries)
Pure maple syrup, for serving

1. In a large bowl, whisk together the almond flour, arrowroot, coconut flour, baking powder, and salt.
2. In a medium bowl, whisk together the almond milk, eggs, ghee, honey, and vanilla.
3. Pour the wet ingredients into the dry ingredients. Stir until the batter comes together. (Add a little more almond milk, if needed to thin the batter.)
4. Spray a large skillet or griddle with olive oil cooking spray and place over medium heat.
5. Drop the batter onto the skillet in 3-inch (7.5 cm) circles. Cook the pancakes for about 2 minutes on each side, or until golden brown on both sides. Remove the pancakes to a plate and cover to keep warm.
6. Meanwhile, form the sausage into 3-inch (7.5 cm) patties.
7. Add the olive oil to the same skillet and increase the heat to medium-high.
8. Add the sausage patties. Cook until the internal temperature reaches 160°F (71°C), about 5 minutes on each side. Remove to a paper towel-lined plate to drain excess oil.
9. Assemble the sliders by placing 1 pancake on the bottom with a sausage patty in the middle, with another pancake on top to make a sandwich.
10. Garnish with the mixed berries and drizzle with maple syrup.

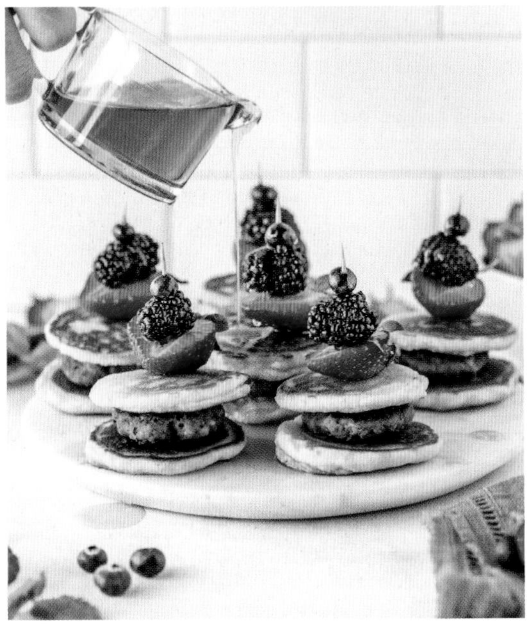

Chocolate-Covered Frozen Banana Bites

What are you going to do when your kids are in the background screaming for a snack? I have an idea: Be the hero and have these banana bites—smeared with nut butter and covered in dark chocolate and crushed almonds—ready in the freezer. They're just sweet enough and are perfect nibbles, no matter what time of year it is.

TRADITIONAL PALEO

Makes: 22 to 25 bites / **Prep Time:** 15 to 20 minutes / **Total Time:** 4 hours

---

3 or 4 bananas, sliced ¼ inch (6 mm) thick

¼ cup (60 g) almond or cashew butter

Toothpicks

10 ounces (280 g) 85% or higher dark chocolate, chopped

2 tablespoons (30 ml) coconut oil

⅓ cup (50 g) almonds

---

1. Line a baking sheet that can fit in the freezer with parchment paper.
2. Lay the banana slices on top of the parchment paper. Evenly coat the top of half the banana slices with the nut butter and top with another banana slice.
3. Insert a toothpick into the middle of each sandwich (this will make it easier to dip in the chocolate). Transfer the banana sandwiches to the freezer for 2 hours.
4. Once the bananas are frozen, add the chocolate and coconut oil to a microwave-safe bowl. Heat for 30 seconds, stir, and repeat until melted.
5. Add the almonds to a food processor and process until finely ground. Transfer to a small bowl.
6. Remove the baking sheet from the freezer and dip the banana stacks, one at a time, into the warm chocolate until completely covered. Dip in the crushed almonds and return to the parchment paper.
7. When all the bananas are dipped, return them to the freezer for 2 more hours.
8. Store in a freezer-safe container.

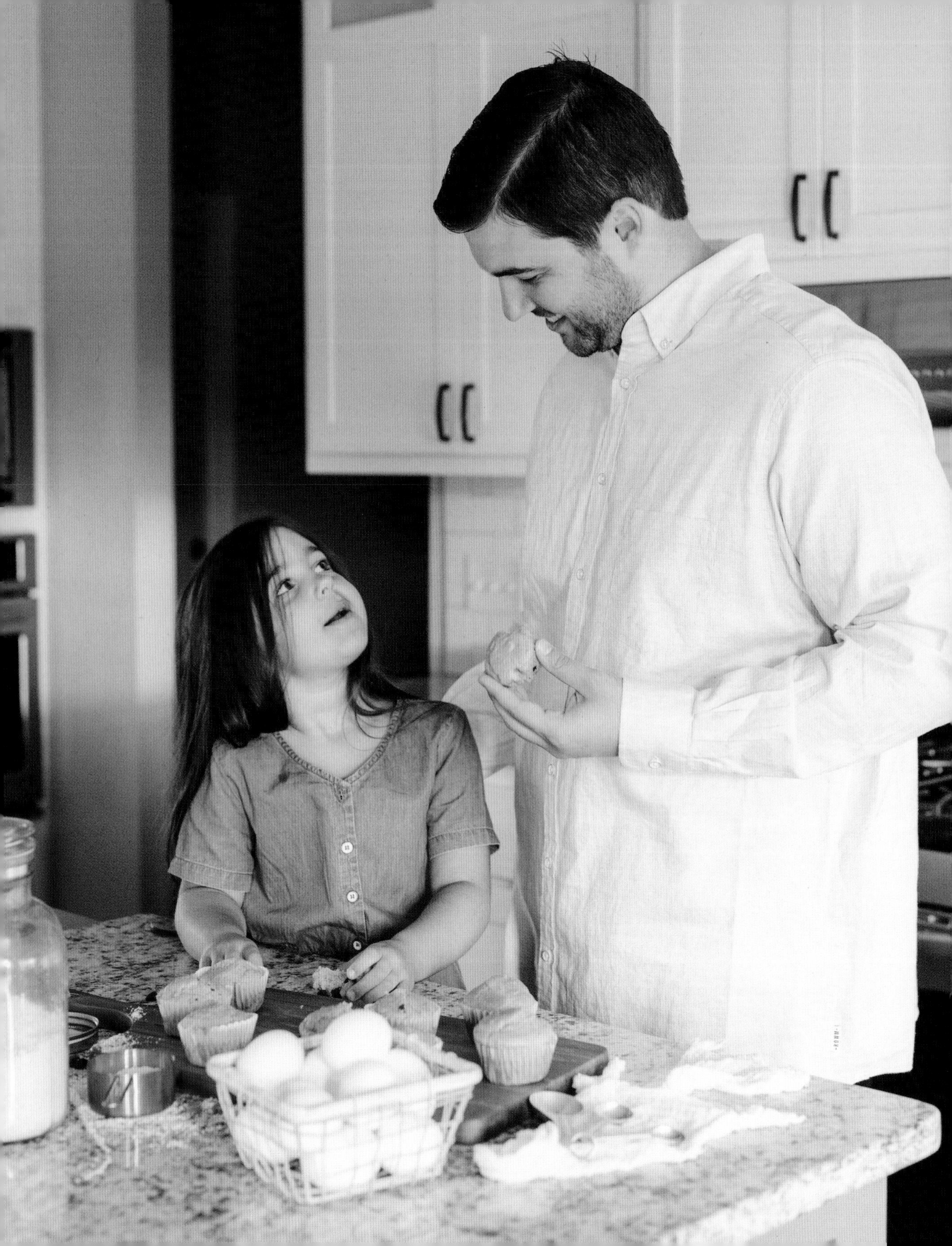

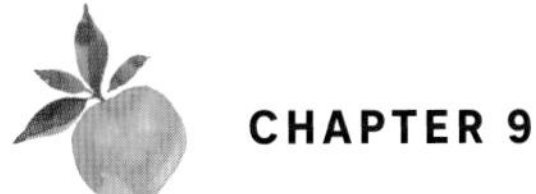

CHAPTER 9

Sweet Treats and Drinks

There are two ways to my heart: muffins and hugs! Yes, that's correct–I don't need diamonds to be happy, just give me food. I have a big sweet tooth, and I love creating healthy Paleo desserts that satisfy my whole family's sweet tooth cravings. You won't even believe these desserts are made with clean and wholesome ingredients. They are rich, decadent, and family approved.

In addition to sweets, I love a good mocktail and smoothie. The creamy Mixed Berry Smoothie (page 182) and refreshing Orange and Thyme Mocktail (page 181) in this chapter are at the very top of my list.

Banana Cream Pie Pops

Growing up, banana cream pie was my favorite dessert. This ice-pop recipe plays on that, and it's perfect for all you banana lovers out there. Ice pops are a great way to tame a sweet tooth in a healthy and cool way.

TRADITIONAL PALEO

Makes: 6 pops / **Prep Time:** 3 minutes / **Total Time:** 10 minutes + 2 hours freeze time

1 whole banana
1 can (13.5 ounces [378 g]) unsweetened coconut milk
5 tablespoons (75 ml) sweetener of choice (I use maple syrup)
1 teaspoon pure vanilla extract
Pinch of sea salt
½ banana, sliced
6 ice-pops molds
⅓ cup (45 g) almonds
¼ cup (60 ml) pure maple syrup

1. Add the whole banana, coconut milk, sweetener, vanilla, and salt to a blender and blend until combined and smooth.
2. Place a couple of banana slices into each ice-pop mold.
3. Pour the creamy mixture into each ice-pop mold. Do not overfill it or the mixture will spill out the sides when putting on the lid.
4. Freeze until completely frozen, 2 to 3 hours.
5. Add the almonds to a food processor and pulse until ground.
6. Pour the maple syrup into a small bowl.
7. Remove the pops from the freezer and unmold. (You might have to quickly run them under warm water to loosen.)
8. Dip the tips of each pop into the maple syrup and then into the crushed almonds.
9. Serve immediately or return the ice pops to the freezer.

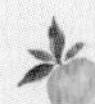

RECIPE NOTES

Ice pops will keep for 3 or 4 weeks (without the syrup and almonds) if stored in an airtight container.

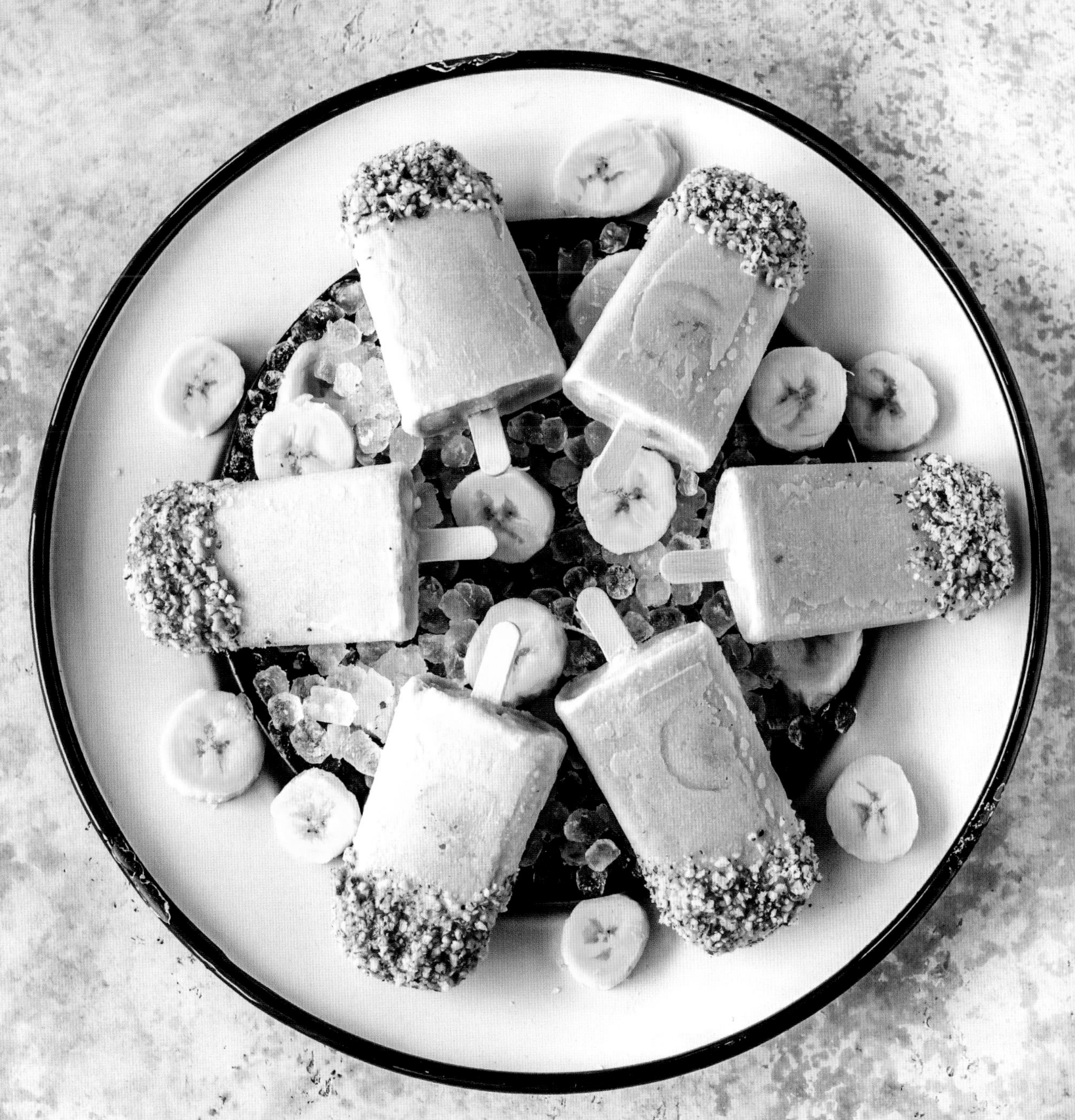

Lemon and Blueberry Cookies

This is the perfect cookie for when your cookie monster mood strikes. It's light and lemony and just sweet enough.

KETO PALEO / TRADITIONAL PALEO

Makes: 12 to 14 cookies / **Prep Time:** 10 to 15 minutes / **Total Time:** 25 to 30 minutes

COOKIES

2 cups (192 g) almond flour
3 tablespoons (18 g) coconut flour
½ teaspoon baking soda + ½ teaspoon cream of tartar
¼ teaspoon sea salt
1 large egg
½ cup (120 g) coconut oil, melted
½ cup (120 ml) pure maple syrup
2 tablespoons (30 ml) lemon juice
1 teaspoon lemon extract
1 teaspoon lemon zest, plus more for garnish
½ teaspoon pure vanilla extract
½ cup (75 g) blueberries

GLAZE

2 tablespoons (28 g) coconut butter
½ cup (120 ml) coconut cream
2 ½ tablespoons (37 ml) monk fruit syrup or maple syrup
2 teaspoons lemon juice
½ teaspoon lemon zest

COOKIES

1. Preheat the oven to 350°F (180°C or gas mark 4) and line a baking sheet with parchment paper.
2. In a medium bowl, whisk together the almond flour, coconut flour, baking powder, and salt.
3. In a large bowl, whisk together the egg, coconut oil, maple syrup, lemon juice, lemon extract, lemon zest, and vanilla.
4. Add the dry ingredients to the wet ingredients and mix until completely combined. Fold in the blueberries.
5. Form the dough into golf ball-size balls and place on the prepared baking sheet, making sure to space them a few inches apart. Gently press down on each ball with the palm of your hand until about 1½ inches (3.8 cm) in diameter.
6. Bake the cookies until browned around the edges and the center is set, 12 to 15 minutes.
7. Remove the cookies from the oven and transfer to a rack to cool completely.
8. Drizzle the cookies with the glaze and sprinkle with the fresh lemon zest.
9. Store in an airtight container for up to 2 weeks. You can also freeze in an airtight container for up to 3 months.

GLAZE

1. Add all the ingredients to a sauce pan. Bring to a boil and then lower the heat and allow to simmer for 5 minutes, stirring occasionally.
2. Transfer the glaze to a small bowl and place in the fridge for 5–10 minutes. The glaze will thicken as it cools.

Double Chocolate Brownies

Brownies that are Paleo compliant and keto? Yes, you can have your brownie and eat it too.

KETO PALEO / TRADITIONAL PALEO

Makes: 12 brownies / **Prep Time:** 5 minutes / **Total Time:** 25 minutes

- 1 cup (96 g) almond flour
- ¾ cup (180 ml) sweetener of choice (see Note)
- ½ cup (60 g) unsweetened cocoa powder
- ¼ teaspoon baking soda + ¼ teaspoon cream of tartar
- ¼ teaspoon sea salt
- 3 large eggs
- ⅓ cup (80 g) ghee, melted
- 3 tablespoons (45 ml) water
- ½ teaspoon pure vanilla extract
- ⅓ cup (58 g) dark chocolate chips (the darker the better)
- ½ teaspoon coarse sea salt

1. Preheat the oven to 350°F (180°C or gas mark 4). Coat an 8 by 8-inch (20 by 20 cm) baking pan with olive oil or cooking spray.
2. In a medium bowl, whisk together the almond flour, sweetener of choice, cocoa powder, baking powder, and salt.
3. In a large bowl, whisk together the eggs, ghee, water, and vanilla.
4. Use a rubber spatula to fold the dry ingredients into the wet ingredients in ¼-cup (30 g) increments. This is to make sure it blends nicely together.
5. Use the spatula to scrape the sides of the bowl and transfer the batter evenly to the prepared baking dish.
6. Bake until the desired doneness, 20 to 25 minutes. I usually bake mine for 21 minutes for a gooey texture. If you like your brownies firmer, I suggest baking for 24 minutes.
7. Allow to cool completely before cutting.
8. Melt the chocolate chips in the microwave in 30-second increments, stirring in between. Drizzle with a spoon over the brownies and sprinkle with the coarse salt.
9. Store any extras in an airtight container for up to 1 week.

RECIPE NOTES

For Keto Paleo, use monk fruit; for Traditional Paleo, use coconut sugar.

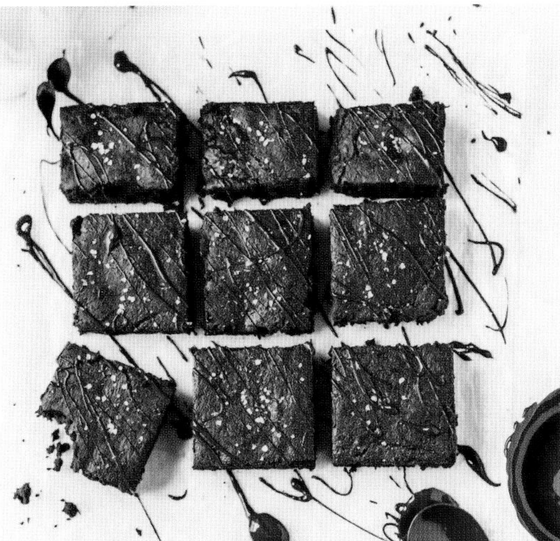

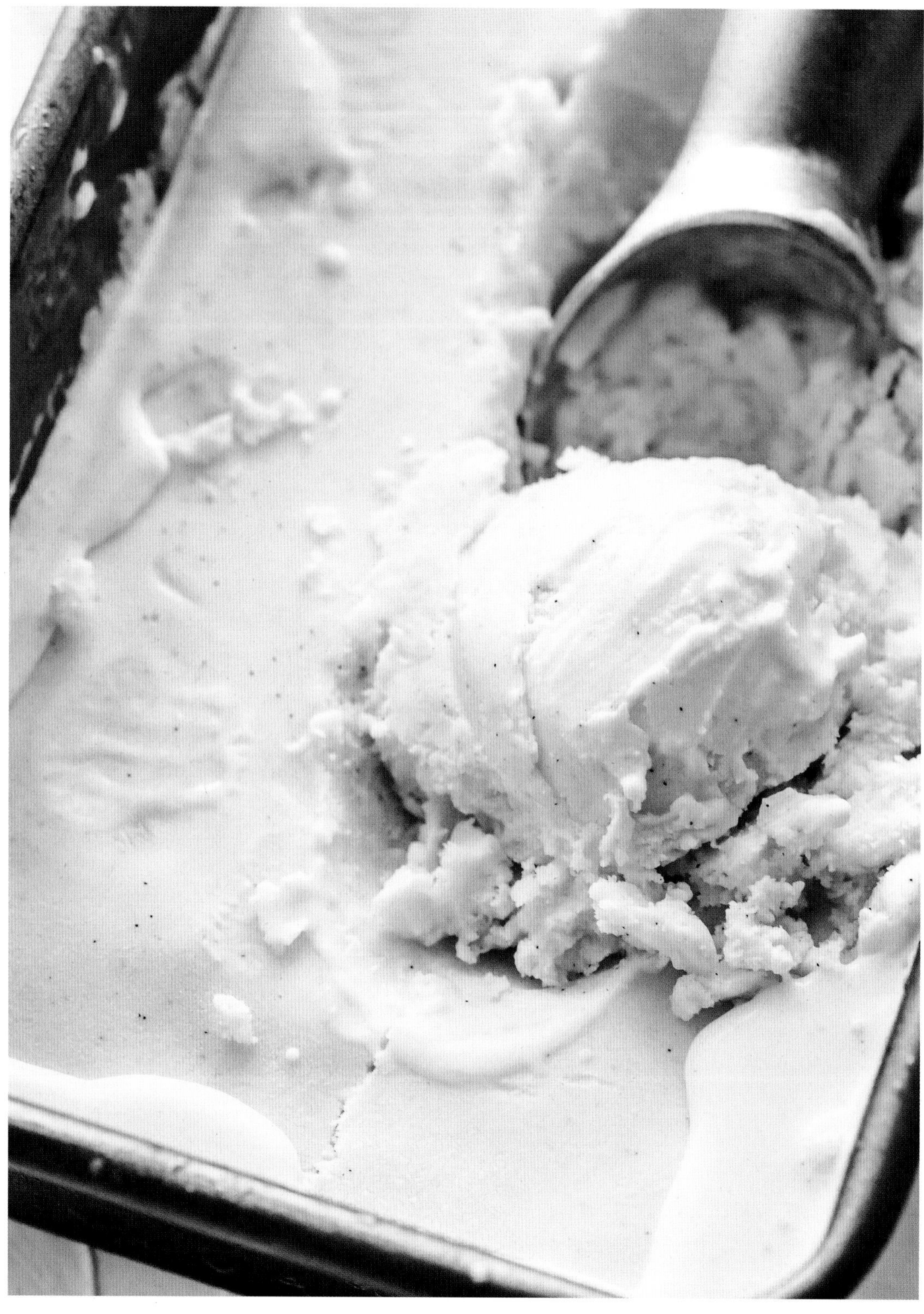

Vanilla Bean Ice Cream

You scream. I scream. We all scream for ice cream! Serve this dairy-free ice cream over Peach Crisp (page 174), with a Double Chocolate Brownie (page 167), or just with a spoon. And don't worry if you don't have an ice cream maker; you can still make this frozen treat.

TRADITIONAL PALEO / KETO PALEO

Makes: 6 servings / **Prep Time:** 5 minutes / **Total Time:** 35 minutes + freezing time

1 vanilla bean
2 cans (13.5 ounces [378 g]) unsweetened coconut milk, chilled
½ cup (120 ml) natural sweetener of choice (I use monk fruit)
1 teaspoon pure vanilla extract
1 teaspoon tapioca flour or arrowroot powder

CHURN VERSION

1. One hour before making the ice cream, put the ice cream canister in the freezer to chill.
2. On a cutting board, use a sharp paring knife to split the vanilla bean lengthwise. Run the edge of the knife along the cut sides of the bean to scrape out the seeds. Transfer the seeds to a high-speed blender.
3. Add the coconut milk, sweetener, vanilla, and tapioca. Blend on high speed until smooth and combined.
4. Transfer the mixture to the chilled canister and follow the instructions for your ice cream maker. All ice cream makers are not the same, so be sure to follow the instructions for your machine.
5. Transfer the mixture to a freezer-safe container and freeze for 5 to 6 hours.
6. Before serving, allow the ice cream to sit out for 5 to 10 minutes so it's easier to scoop.

NO-CHURN VERSION

1. Follow the instructions for churning through step 3.
2. Add the liquid ice cream mixture to a freezer-safe container and put in the freezer.
3. Freeze until firm, 5 to 6 hours. Remove the ice cream a couple of times during the 5 to 6 hours and mix with a spoon.
4. Before serving, allow the ice cream to sit out for 5 to 10 minutes so it's easier to scoop.

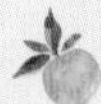

RECIPE NOTES

For Keto, replace the tapioca with ⅛ teaspoon xanthan gum or 1½ teaspoons gelatin.

Chocolate Chip Muffins

Chocolate chip cookies are out, and these Paleo chocolate chip muffins are in. Make a batch (or two) at the beginning of the week and enjoy as a grab-and-go breakfast or as an afternoon treat.

KETO PALEO / TRADITIONAL PALEO

Makes: 10 to 12 muffins / **Prep Time:** 5 to 7 minutes / **Total Time:** 35 minutes

- 2½ cups (240 g) almond flour
- ½ teaspoon baking soda + ½ teaspoon cream of tartar
- ¼ teaspoon sea salt
- 3 large eggs, at room temperature
- ½ cup (170 g) honey or sweetener of choice (see Note)
- 2½ tablespoons (37 ml) canned unsweetened coconut milk
- 3 tablespoons (28 g) ghee or coconut oil, melted
- 1 teaspoon pure vanilla extract
- ⅓ cup (58 g) dark chocolate chips

1. Preheat the oven to 350°F (180°C or gas mark 4) and line a cupcake pan with 12 paper liners.
2. In a medium bowl, whisk together the almond flour, baking powder, and salt.
3. In a large bowl, whisk together the eggs, honey, coconut milk, ghee, and vanilla.
4. Use a rubber spatula to fold the dry ingredients into the wet ingredients in ¼-cup (30 g) increments. Fold in the chocolate chips.
5. Spoon the batter evenly into the paper liners.
6. Bake until a toothpick inserted into the center of a muffin comes out clean, 18 to 20 minutes.
7. Let the muffins cool in the pan for 5 to 10 minutes before serving.
8. Store in an airtight container at room temperature for up to 2 weeks. Will keep inthe freezer in an airtight freezer-proof container for 2 to 3 months.

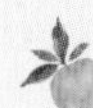

RECIPE NOTES

Use monk fruit for Keto Paleo and honey for Traditional Paleo.

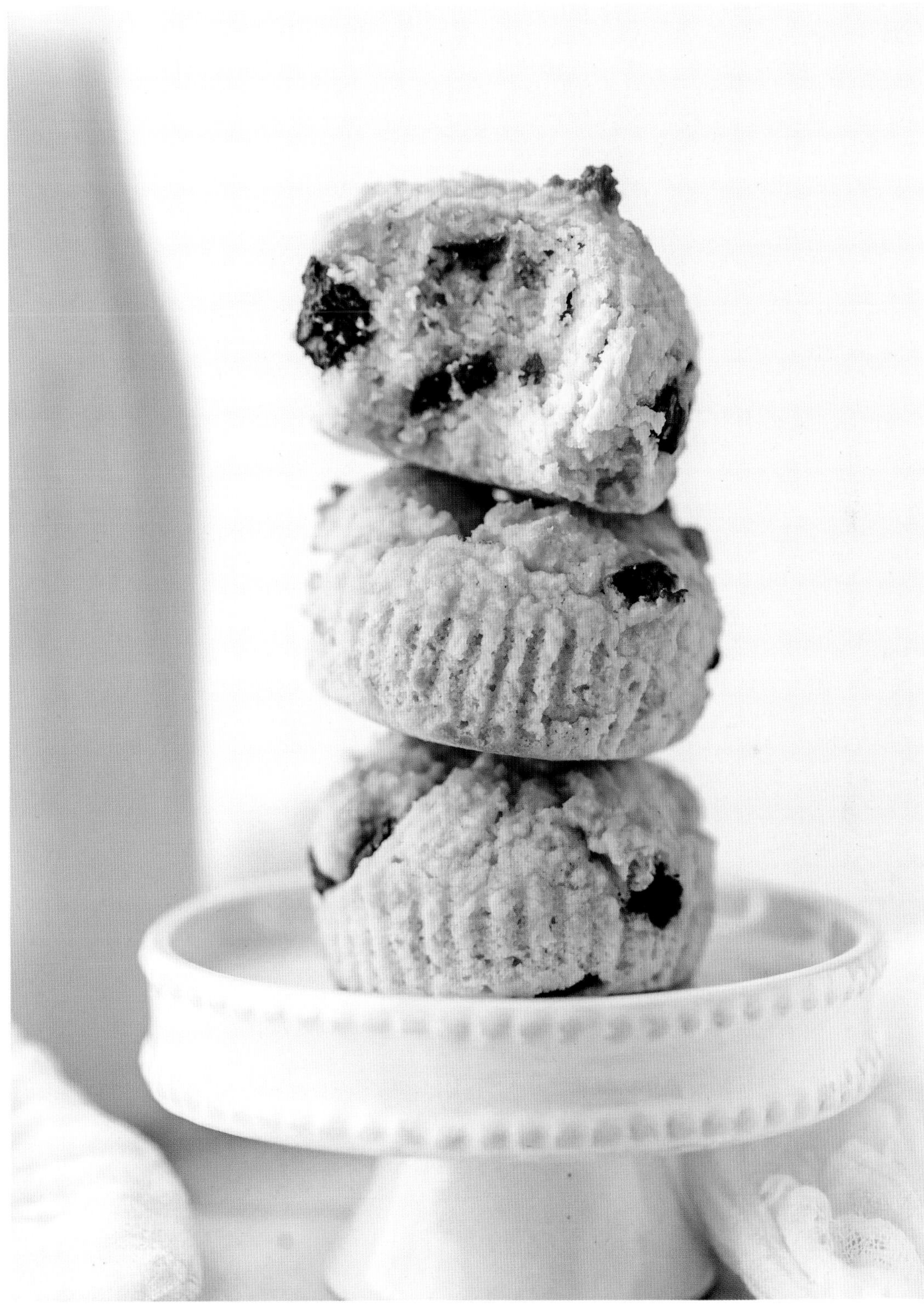

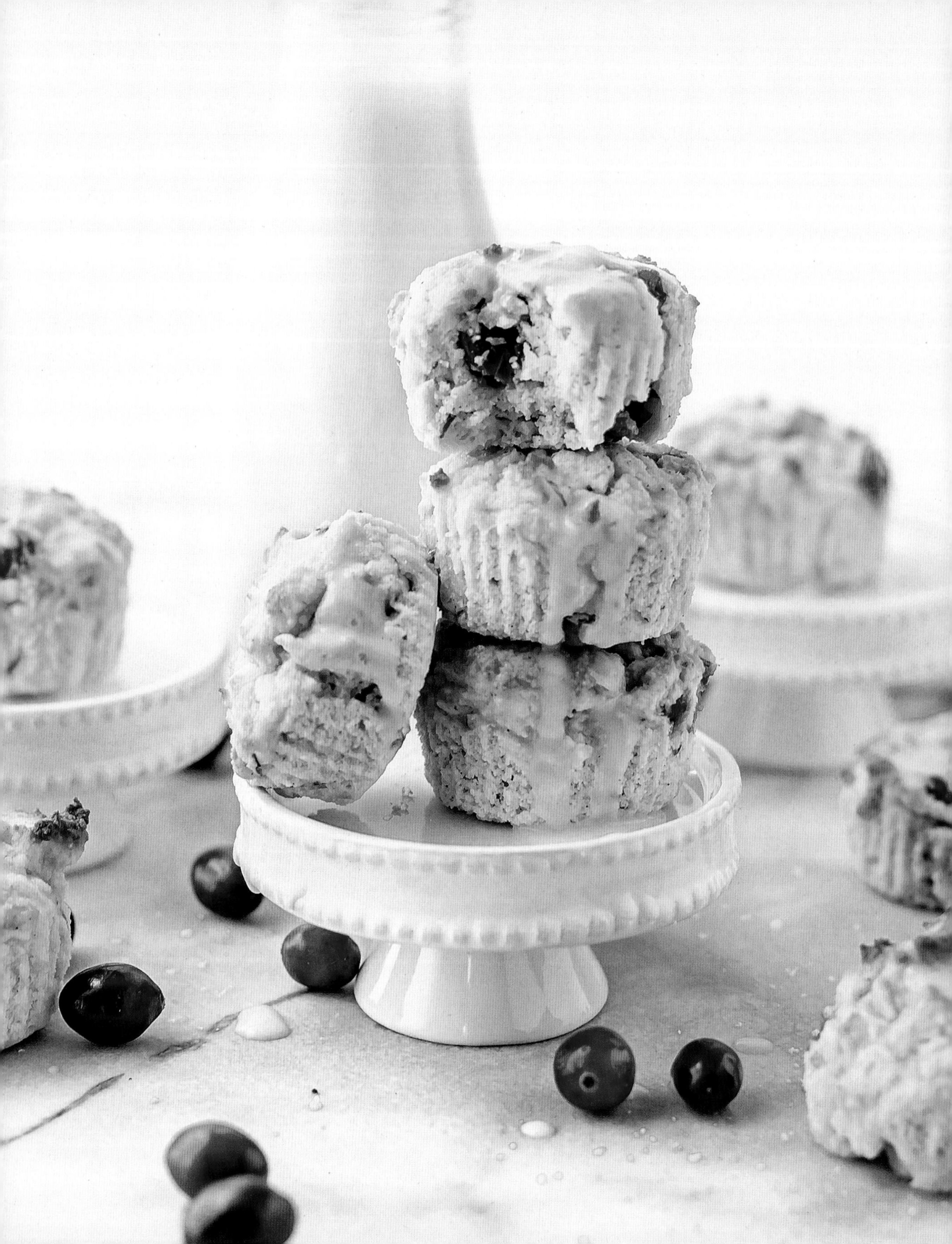

Cranberry-Orange Muffins

Cranberries aren't just for the holidays! They can be used year-round to make sweet treats such as these Paleo muffins that are bursting with bright flavor.

TRADITIONAL PALEO

Makes: 10 to 12 muffins / **Prep Time:** 5 to 10 minutes / **Total Time:** 35 minutes

MUFFINS

2½ cups (240 g) almond flour
½ cup (48 g) tapioca flour
½ teaspoon baking soda + ½ teaspoon cream of tartar
3 large eggs, at room temperature
⅓ cup (113 g) honey or sweetener of choice
3½ tablespoons (52 ml) fresh squeezed orange juice
2½ tablespoons (35 g) coconut oil or ghee, melted
1 tablespoon (15 ml) canned unsweetened coconut milk
1 tablespoon (6 g) orange zest
¼ teaspoon sea salt
½ cup (50 g) fresh or frozen cranberries

GLAZE

2 tablespoons (28 g) coconut butter
½ cup (120 ml) coconut cream
2 ½ tablespoons (37 ml) monk fruit syrup or maple syrup
2 teaspoons orange juice
½ teaspoon orange zest

MUFFINS

1. Preheat the oven to 350°F (180°C or gas mark 4) and line a cupcake pan with 12 paper liners.
2. In a medium bowl, whisk together the almond flour, tapioca flour, and baking powder.
3. In a large bowl, whisk together the eggs, honey, orange juice, coconut oil, coconut milk, orange zest, and salt.
4. Use a rubber spatula to fold the dry ingredients into the wet ingredients in ¼-cup (30 g) increments. Fold in the cranberries
5. Spoon the batter evenly into the paper liners.
6. Bake until a toothpick inserted into the center of a muffin comes out clean, 18 to 20 minutes.
7. Let the muffins cool in the pan for 5 to 10 minutes and then remove from the pan and let cool completely.
8. Drizzle each muffin with the glaze before serving.
9. Store in an airtight container at room temperature for up to 2 weeks. Will keep in the freezer in an airtight freezer-proof container for 2 to 3 months.

GLAZE

1. Add all the ingredients to a sauce pan. Bring to a boil and then lower the heat and allow to simmer for 5 minutes, stirring occasionally.
2. Transfer the glaze to a small bowl and place in the fridge for 5–10 minutes. The glaze will thicken as it cools.

Peach Crisp

If you're feeling peachy and need a sweet treat, you'll love this recipe. I combine fresh peach slices with all-natural sweeteners and bake it topped with a nutty crumble. Add a dollop of creamy Vanilla Bean Ice Cream (page 169), and this fresh recipe is sure to make you smile.

TRADITIONAL PALEO

Makes: 6 servings / **Prep Time:** 15 minutes / **Total Time:** 35 minutes

FILLING

6 peaches, sliced (skin on)
⅓ cup (80 ml) pure maple syrup
2 tablespoons (20 g) coconut sugar
1 tablespoon (20 g) honey
1 tablespoon (6 g) tapioca flour
1 teaspoon lemon juice
½ teaspoon pure vanilla extract

TOPPING

½ cup (75 g) pecans or walnuts
¼ cup (24 g) almond flour
2 tablespoons (40 g) honey
2 tablespoons (28 g) ghee or coconut oil, melted
1 tablespoon (6 g) tapioca flour
1 teaspoon lemon zest
¼ teaspoon sea salt

Vanilla Bean Ice Cream (page 169), for serving (optional)

FILLING

1. Preheat the oven to 350°F (180°C or gas mark 4). Grease a cast-iron skillet or 9 by 9-inch (23 by 23 cm) baking dish of choice.
2. In a large bowl, combine the peaches, maple syrup, coconut sugar, honey, tapioca flour, lemon juice, and vanilla. Mix together with a spoon until well combined.
3. Transfer the filling to the prepared baking vessel.

TOPPING

1. Add the pecans, almond flour, honey, ghee, tapioca flour, lemon zest, and salt to a food processor. Pulse until the mixture is crumbly.
2. Evenly top the peach filling with the crumble topping.
3. Bake until the top is golden and the filling is bubbling, 18 to 20 minutes.
4. Serve hot with a scoop of ice cream, if desired.

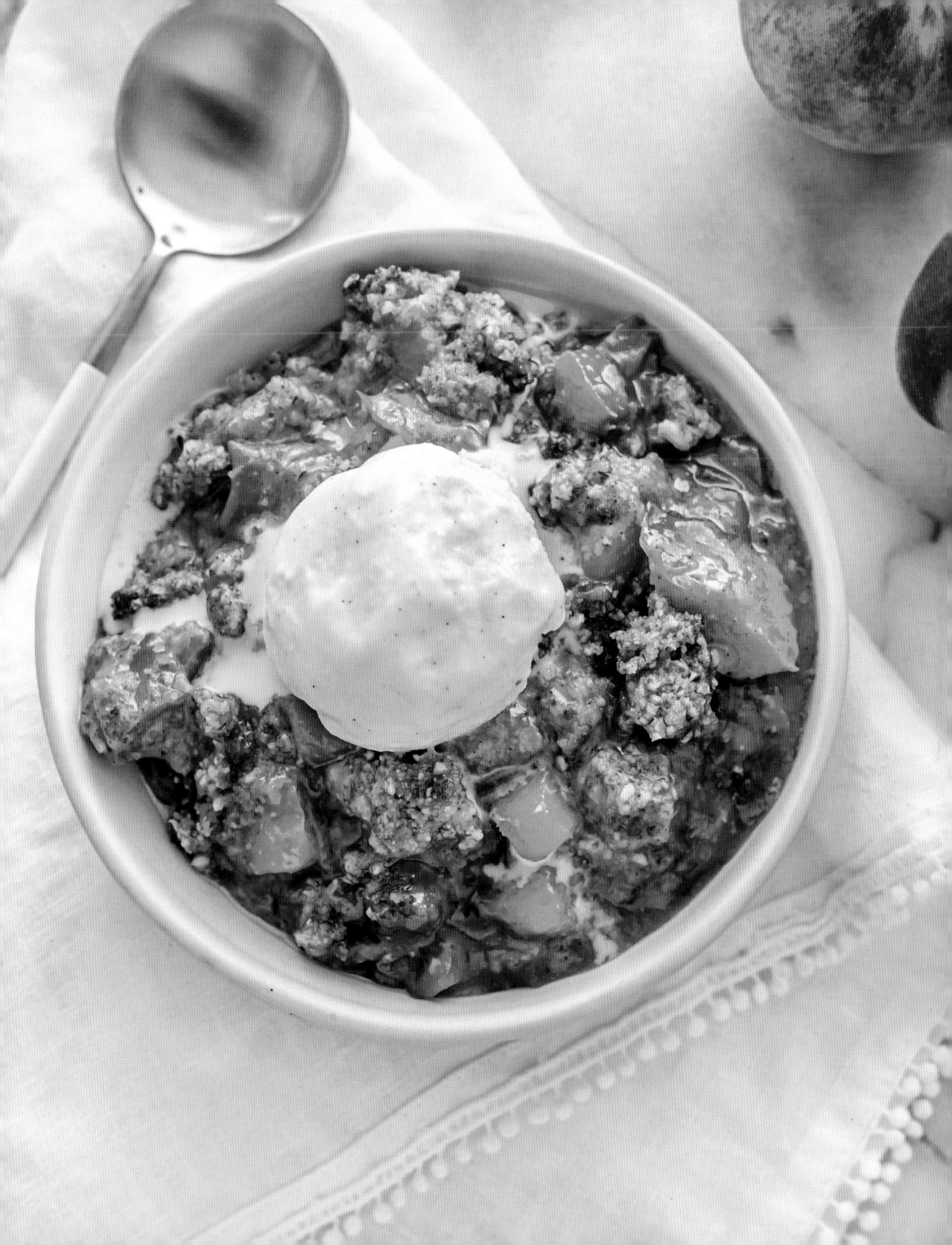

Strawberry Lemonade Bars

Refresh your senses with these frozen strawberry lemonade bars. The chewy, nutty crust topped with a creamy strawberry-lemon filling is great for social gatherings or as a weekend treat for the entire family.

TRADITIONAL PALEO

Makes: 9 to 12 bars / **Prep Time:** 5 minutes / **Total Time:** 15 minutes + 3 hours freeze time

CRUST

¾ cup (135 g) pitted Medjool dates
¾ cup (105 g) almonds
¼ cup (35 g) pecans
¼ cup (20 g) unsweetened shredded coconut
Juice of 1 lemon
1 tablespoon (15 ml) pure maple syrup
1 teaspoon lemon zest
½ teaspoon pure vanilla extract

FILLING

1 can (13.5 ounces [378 g]) unsweetened coconut milk, chilled
½ cup (75 g) fresh or frozen strawberries
3½ tablespoons (70 g) honey or sweetener of choice
Juice of 1 lemon
2 tablespoons (12 g) tapioca flour
1 tablespoon (14 g) soft coconut oil
1 teaspoon pure vanilla extract
Zest of ½ lemon

CRUST

1. Line an 8 by 8-inch (20 by 20 cm) baking dish with parchment paper.
2. Add the dates, almonds, pecans, coconut, lemon juice, maple syrup, lemon zest, and vanilla to a food processor. Pulse until it resembles a crumbly crust.
3. Transfer the crust to the baking dish and spread out evenly by pressing down to form the crust on top of the parchment paper.
4. Put the baking dish in the freezer for 10 minutes.

FILLING

1. Add the coconut milk, strawberries, honey, lemon juice, tapioca flour, coconut oil, vanilla, and lemon zest to a blender. Blend on high speed until smooth.
2. Remove the baking dish from the freezer and pour the filling over the top.
3. Return the dish to the freezer until the bars harden, at least 3 to 4 hours.
4. Remove from the freezer and thaw a little before cutting into bars as desired.

Cinnamon Bun Energy Bites

These healthy, yet crave-worthy, cinnamon bun–flavored nut balls are perfect for mid-morning or afternoon snacking to help get you over the slump. They'll keep you feeling full and energized for hours.

TRADITIONAL PALEO

Makes: 12 balls / **Prep Time:** 5 minutes / **Total Time:** 10 minutes + chill time

- 2 cups walnuts or pecans
- ⅓ cup chopped dates (around 8 whole dates)
- ¼ cup almond flour
- 3 tablespoons maple syrup
- 1 tablespoon ghee or coconut oil, melted
- 1½ teaspoons ground cinnamon
- ¼ teaspoon nutmeg
- 1 teaspoon pure vanilla
- Pinch of salt

COATING

- 2 tablespoons coconut flour
- 1¾ tablespoons coconut sugar
- ¾ teaspoon ground cinnamon

1. Line a baking sheet with parchment paper.
2. In a large food processor, pulse the pecans or walnuts until crumbly.
3. Add the dates, almond flour, maple syrup, ghee or coconut oil, cinnamon, vanilla, and salt. Blend together until it reaches a dough-like consistency. Add more maple syrup or almond flour if needed.
4. In a separate small bowl, add all the coating ingredients and combine.
5. Use a small ice cream scoop to form balls the size of golf ball and roll in the coating and place on the baking sheet.
6. Refrigerate for at least 1 hour before serving or enjoy at room temperature. Store in a glass container in the fridge for up to 1 week.

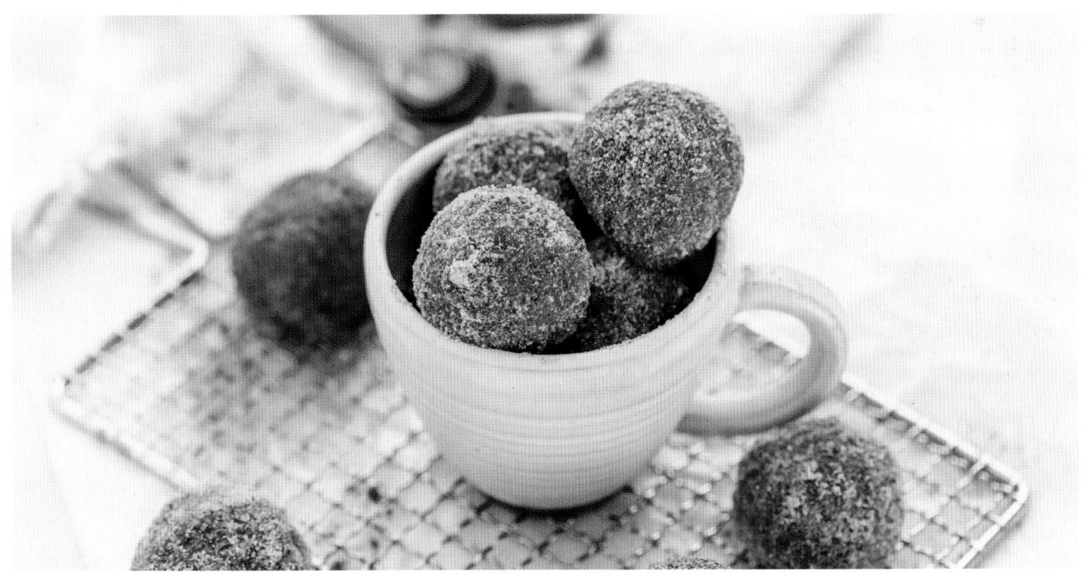

Paleo Banana Bread

This perfect Paleo banana bread is moist and filling. If you are looking for a special morning treat to enjoy with your cup of black coffee, look no further.

TRADITIONAL PALEO

Makes: 10 to 12 servings / **Prep Time:** 5 to 10 minutes / **Total Time:** 50 to 60 minutes

---

2 cups (192 g) almond flour
½ cup (48 g) coconut flour
⅓ cup (80 ml) monk fruit or sweetener of choice
2 teaspoons Paleo baking powder (1 teaspoon baking soda + 1 teaspoon cream of tartar)
1 teaspoon ground cinnamon
Pinch of sea salt
3 brown or very ripe bananas, peeled and smashed
3 large eggs
3 tablespoons (42 g) coconut oil or ghee, melted
1½ teaspoons pure vanilla extract
1 banana, sliced, of preferred ripeness, for top

---

1. Preheat the oven to 350°F (180°C or gas mark 4) and line an 8 by 5-inch (20 by 12.5 cm) loaf pan with parchment paper.
2. In a medium bowl, whisk together the almond flour, coconut flour, monk fruit, baking powder, cinnamon, and salt.
3. In a large bowl, whisk together the bananas, eggs, coconut oil, and vanilla.
4. Carefully fold the dry ingredients into the wet ingredients until combined.
5. Pour the batter into the prepared loaf pan and top with banana slices. Bake until the top is golden brown and the middle is set, 50 to 60 minutes.
6. Allow to cool before slicing. Store in an airtight container for up to 2 weeks. Can also be frozen in an airtight container for up to 3 months.

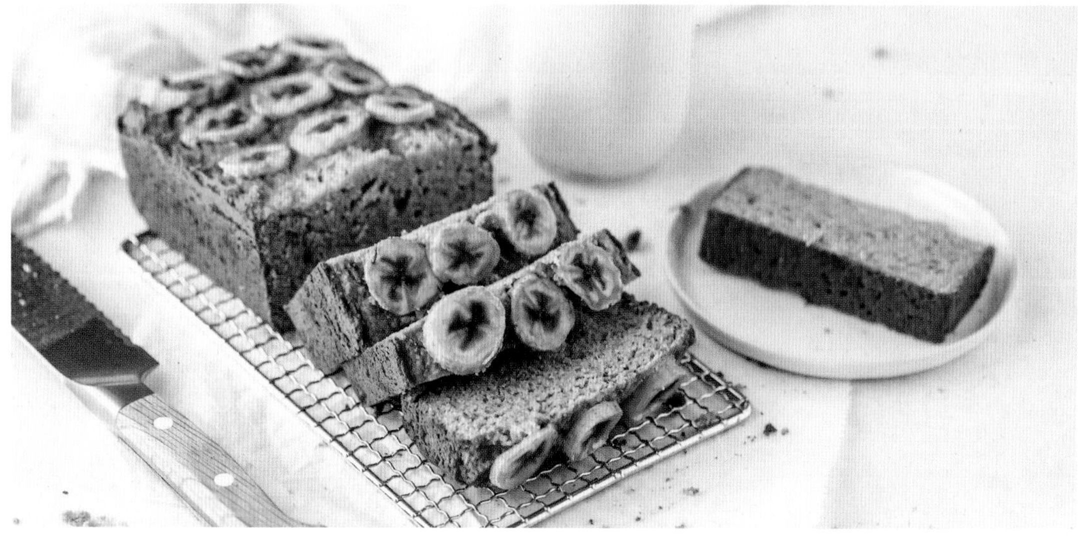

Frozen Fruit Whip

This frozen Paleo fruit whip serves as a refreshing and fruity soft serve dessert. Enjoy during those hot summer months or just as an afternoon treat.

TRADITIONAL PALEO

Makes: 4 servings / **Prep Time:** 2 minutes / **Total Time:** 5 minutes

1 pound (454 g) frozen fruit of choice
¾ cup (180 ml) unsweetened coconut or almond milk (coconut milk will provide a creamier whip)
¼ cup (60 ml) no-sugar-added pineapple juice
1 teaspoon lemon juice
½ teaspoon pure vanilla extract
1 tablespoon (20 g) honey or sweetener of choice (optional)

1. Add the frozen fruit, almond milk, pineapple juice, lemon juice, and vanilla to a high-speed blender and blend until it becomes a sorbet consistency. To get the desired consistency, you may need to add more milk.
2. Taste it and add the honey, if desired, for additional sweetness.
3. Serve immediately or store in the freezer for later enjoyment.

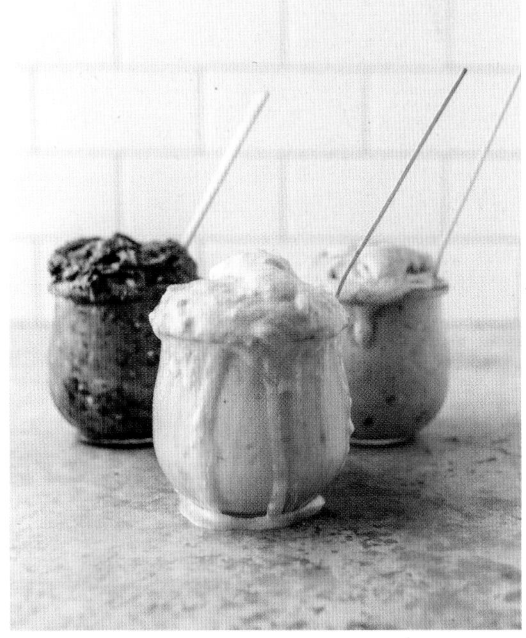

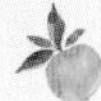

RECIPE NOTES

Store in a freezer-safe container for up to 3 months. Before serving, set the container out at room temperature for 10 minutes. Add the frozen mixture to a blender and rewhip.

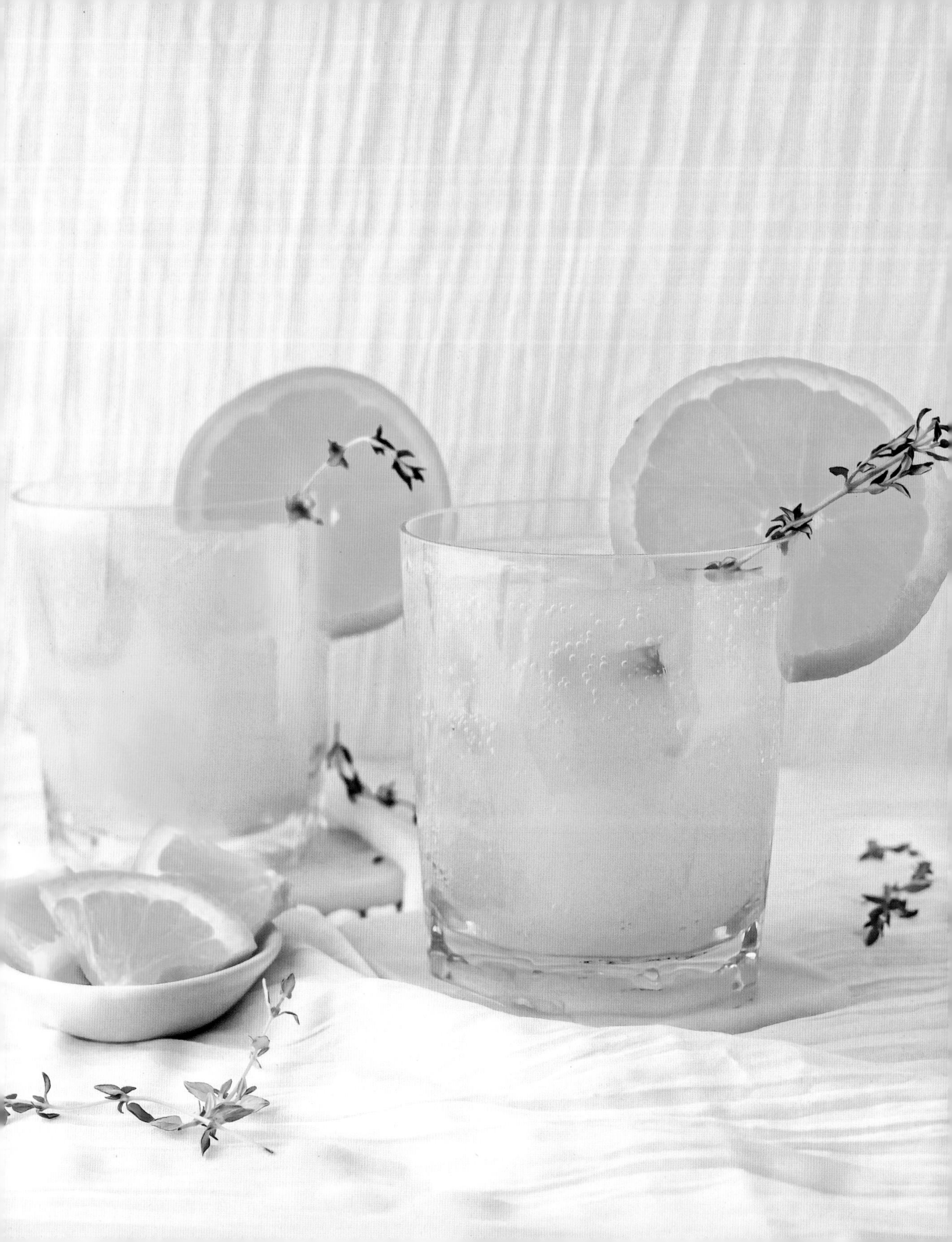

Orange and Thyme Mocktail

Who needs bubbly champagne when you have this crisp and refreshing citrusy mocktail? Cheers!

SQUEAKY CLEAN PALEO / TRADITIONAL PALEO

Makes: 1 drink / **Prep Time:** 3 minutes / **Total Time:** 5 minutes

- ¾ cup (180 ml) sparkling water
- ¼ cup (60 ml) fresh squeezed orange juice
- ¼ cup (60 ml) no-sugar-added pineapple juice
- 1 teaspoon lemon juice
- Ice cubes
- Thyme sprig and orange slice, for garnish

1. In a glass, stir together the sparkling water, orange juice, pineapple juice, and lemon juice.
2. Add ice and garnish with a sprig of thyme and a slice of orange.

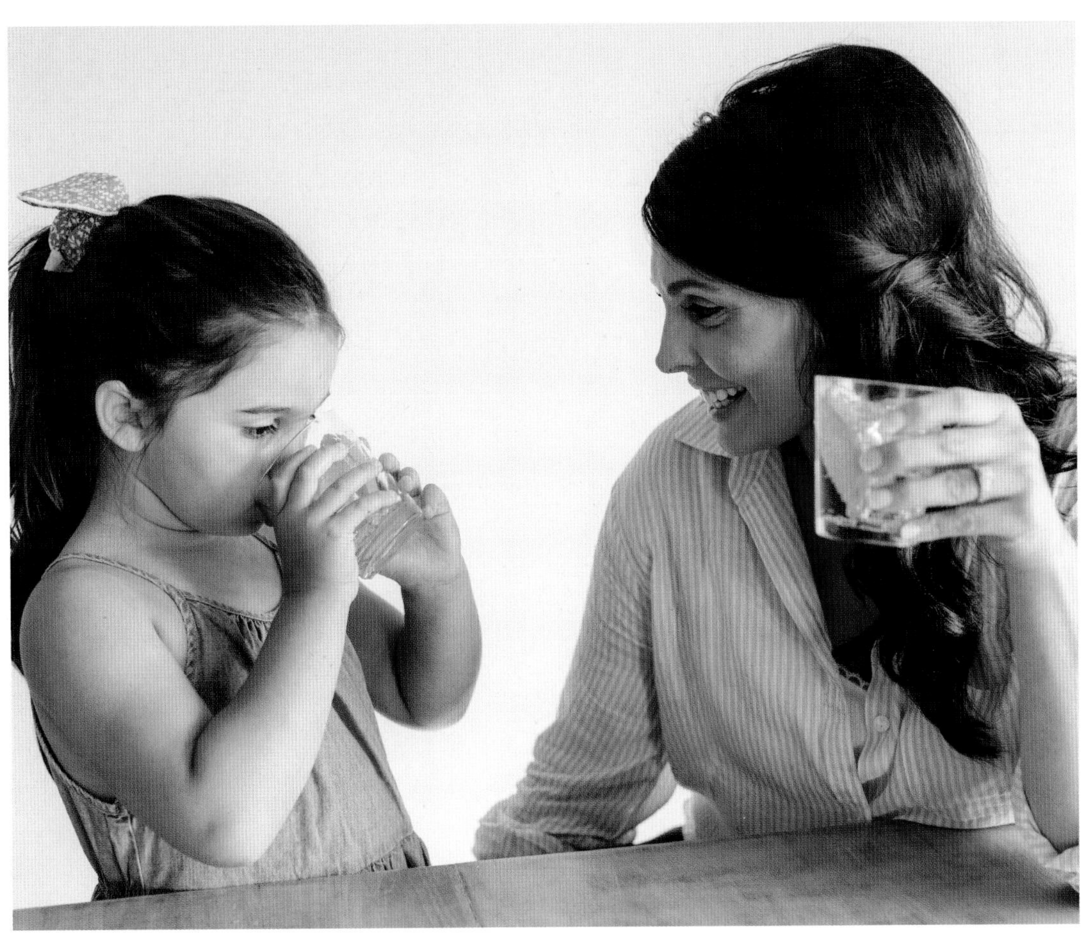

Mixed Berry Smoothie

Whether you're looking for a delicious lower-sugar smoothie or a quick breakfast or kid snack option, this is your recipe.

KETO PALEO / TRADITIONAL PALEO

Makes: 1 smoothie / **Prep Time:** 3 minutes / **Total Time:** 5 minutes

1 cup (240 ml) unsweetened almond milk
¾ cup (120 g) frozen mixed berries (any combination)
2 tablespoons (30 ml) monk fruit or (40 g) honey (see Note)
1 teaspoon pure lemon juice
1 teaspoon pure vanilla extract
½ teaspoon lemon zest

1. Add the almond milk, berries, monk fruit, lemon juice, vanilla, and lemon zest to a blender and blend until smooth and creamy.
2. Enjoy immediately.

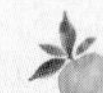

RECIPE NOTES

Use the monk fruit for Keto Paleo and honey for Traditional Paleo.

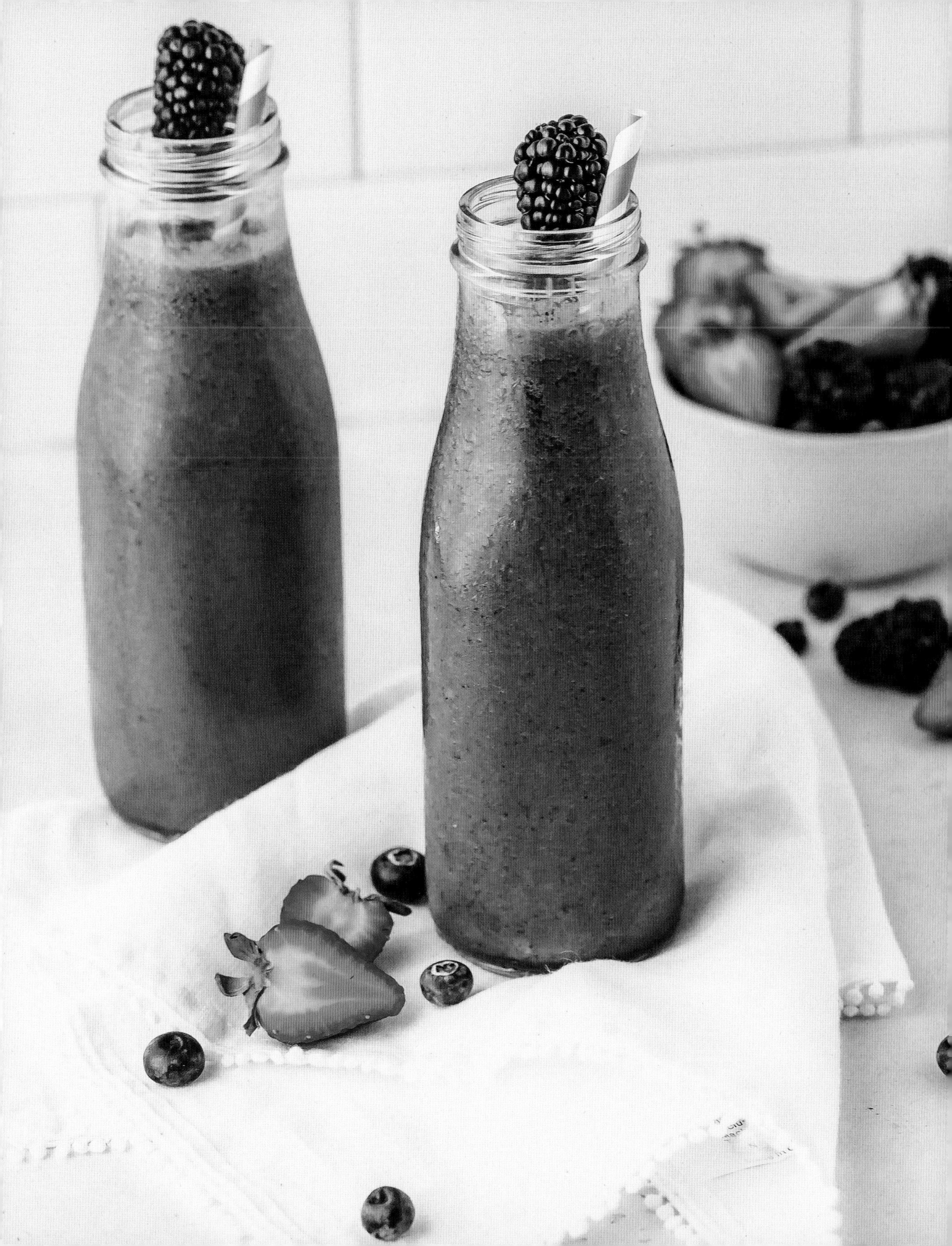

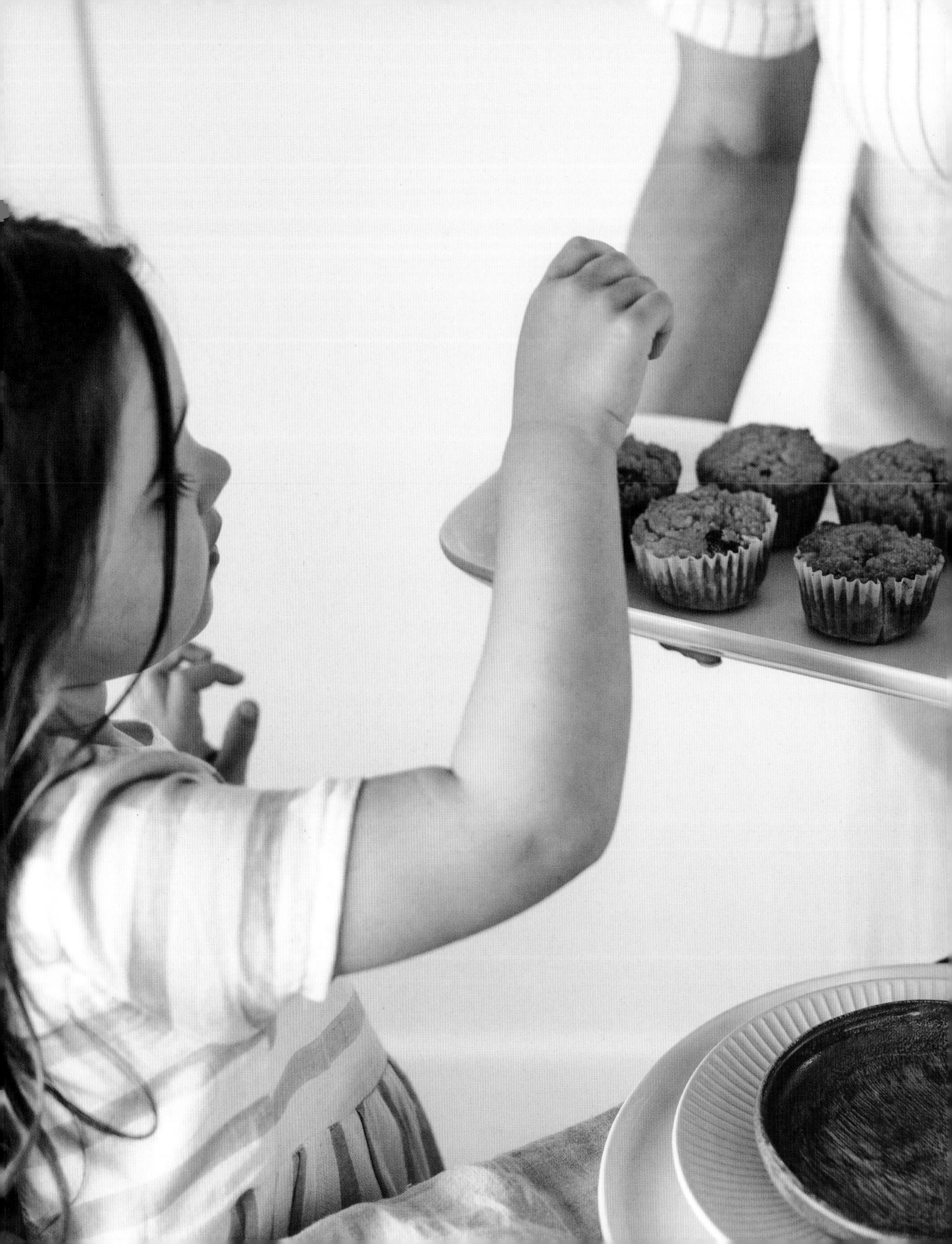

Resources and References

Books

The Bulletproof Diet by David Asprey

Clean Keto vs Dirty Keto by Michael P. Grego D.C., and Kevin Grego

Keto Answers by Anthony Gustin, D.C., M.S., and Chris Irvin, M.S.

The Paleo Cure by Chris Kresser

Wheat Belly by William Davis, M.D.

Websites

Everyday Health | "The Paleo Diet: How It Works, What to Eat, and the Risks"
www.everydayhealth.com/diet-nutrition/the-paleo-diet.aspx

Mayo Clinic | "Paleo diet: What is it and why is it so popular?"
www.mayoclinic.org/healthy-lifestyle/nutrition-and-healthy-eating/in-depth/paleo-diet/art-20111182

The Paleo Diet | Paleo recipes and blogs on a variety of health topics
www.thepaleodiet.com

Perfect Keto | Keto foods and supplements
perfectketo.com

Paleo Leap | Paleo 101
www.paleoleap.com/paleo-101

Whole 30 | Meal plans, podcasts, books, and more resources
www.Whole30.com

About the Author

Ashley McCrary is a recipe creator and the CEO/owner of Healthy Little Peach, a food and lifestyle blog. Her passion is to create healthy recipes that the whole family will love while sharing her real life. Her work has been featured on The Food Network, The Feed, on the Whole30 website, and in Whole30 Friends and Family.

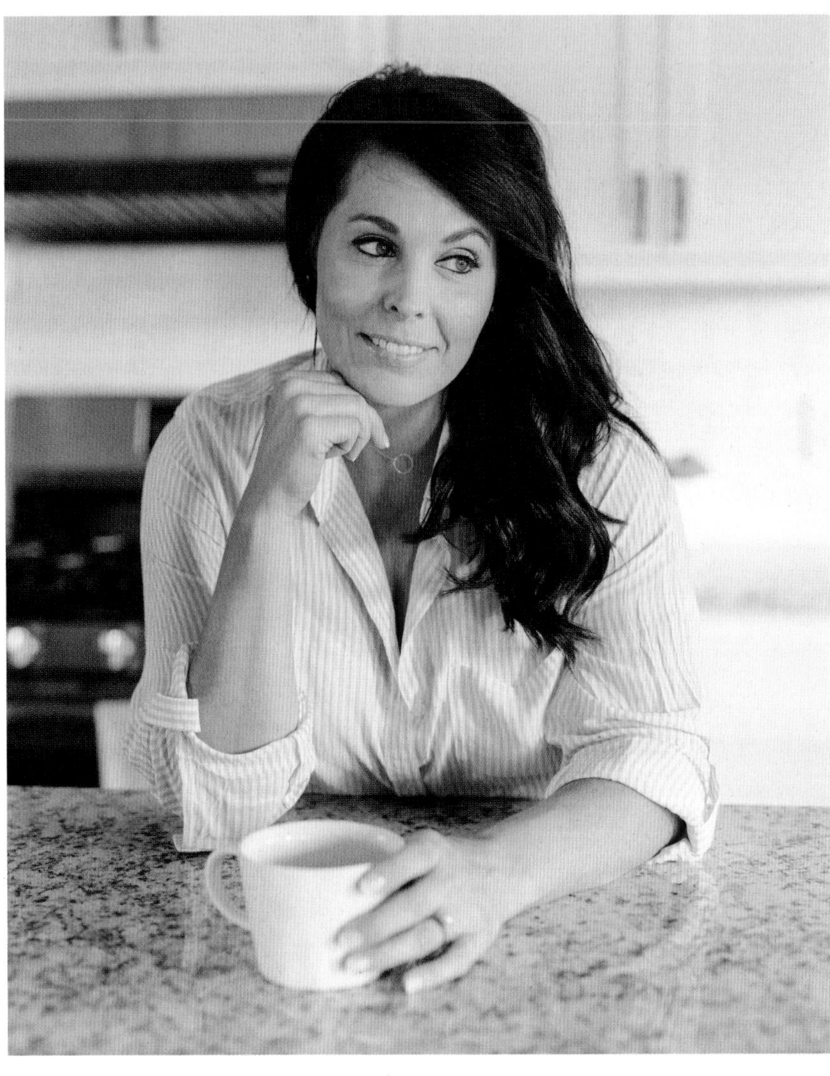

Acknowlegments

This cookbook would not have been possible without the help of my husband Joel; my mother, Tina Michie; and my mother and father-in-law, Randy and Lana McCrary. These precious people stepped up and helped when I needed it the most. I am forever grateful for their support and love.

In addition, I want to thank everyone on the Quarto team. Jill Alexander, my editor and probably one of the sweetest human beings in the world. Thank you for your grace, patience and wisdom. You are truly a gem and I wouldn't have wanted to go through this process with anyone else. My art director, Marissa Giambrone, thank you for helping me bring all my visions to life. And everyone else on the team who was a part of this long but rewarding process. The dedication and commitment that was shown to me was truly amazing.

I want to also thank Grandmother Sue, who always taught me to cook from the heart. Without her guidance and love, I am not sure I would be where I am today. Grandma Sue always said that food is the best way to bring people together and I couldn't agree more. Her motto was cook from the heart, make a mess in the kitchen, and love people in the process.

Lastly, I want to thank my community. Without you guys all of this wouldn't be possible. Thank you all for helping make my dreams come true.

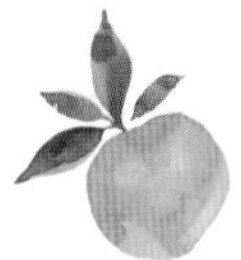

Index

L

M

O

P

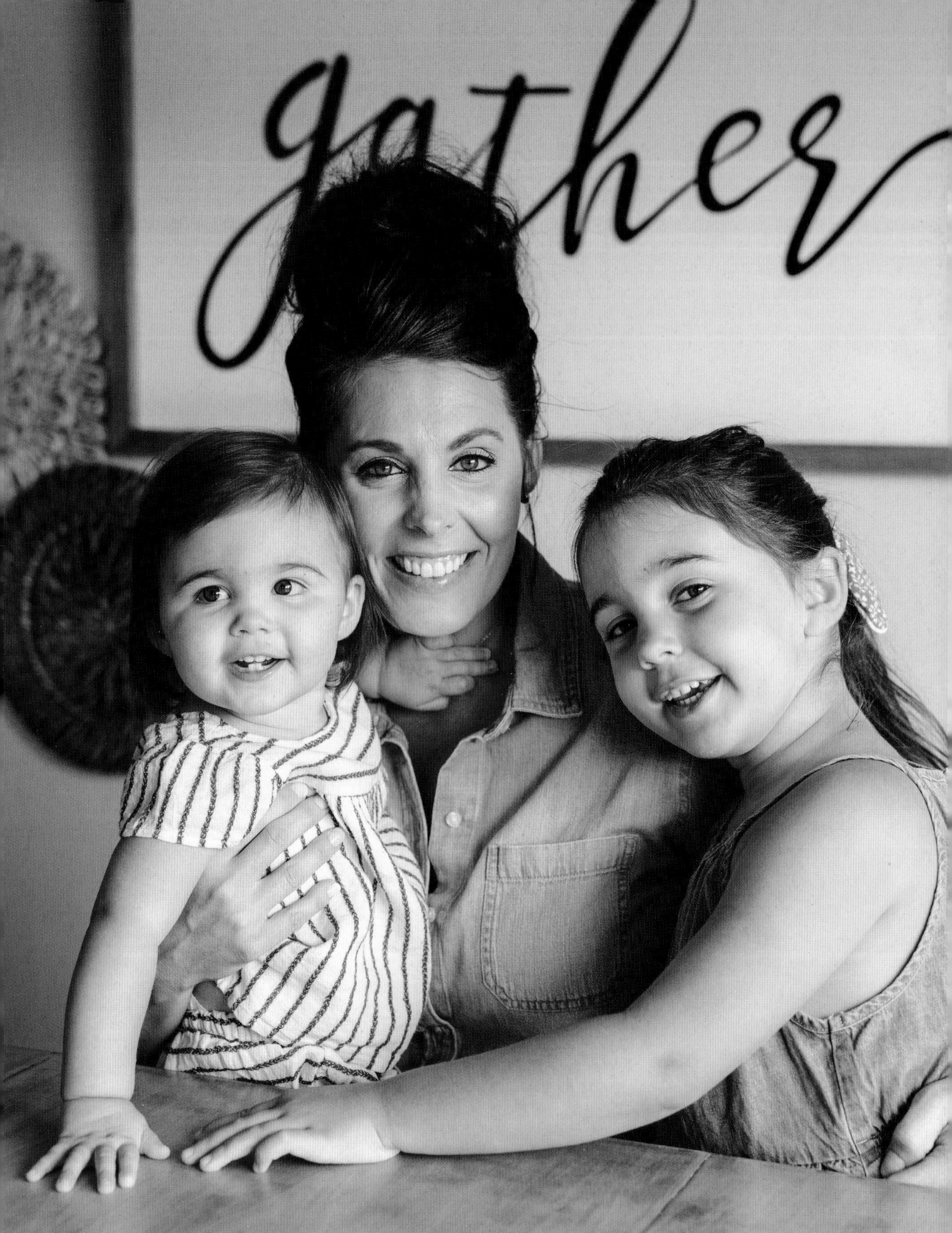
gather